SIMPLE LIFE

(1904)

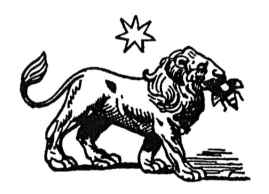

Charles Wagner

ISBN 0-7661-0666-7

Kessinger Publishing's
Rare Mystical Reprints

THOUSANDS OF SCARCE BOOKS
ON THESE AND OTHER SUBJECTS:

Freemasonry * Akashic * Alchemy * Alternative Health * Ancient Civilizations * Anthroposophy * Astrology * Astronomy * Aura * Bible Study * Cabalah * Cartomancy * Chakras * Clairvoyance * Comparative Religions * Divination * Druids * Eastern Thought * Egyptology * Esoterism * Essenes * Etheric * ESP * Gnosticism * Great White Brotherhood * Hermetics * Kabalah * Karma * Knights Templar * Kundalini * Magic * Meditation * Mediumship * Mesmerism * Metaphysics * Mithraism * Mystery Schools * Mysticism * Mythology * Numerology * Occultism * Palmistry * Pantheism * Parapsychology * Philosophy * Prosperity * Psychokinesis * Psychology * Pyramids * Qabalah * Reincarnation * Rosicrucian * Sacred Geometry * Secret Rituals * Secret Societies * Spiritism * Symbolism * Tarot * Telepathy * Theosophy * Transcendentalism * Upanishads * Vedanta * Wisdom * Yoga * *Plus Much More!*

DOWNLOAD A FREE CATALOG AT:
www.kessinger.net

OR EMAIL US AT:
books@kessinger.net

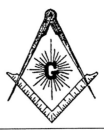

THE SIMPLE LIFE

BY CHARLES WAGNER

Author of The Better Way
By The Fireside

Translated from the French by Mary Louise Hendee

Popular Edition

McClure, Phillips & Co.
New York
1904

COPYRIGHT, 1901, BY
McCLURE, PHILLIPS & CO.

CONTENTS

		PAGE
I.	OUR COMPLEX LIFE . . .	1
II.	THE ESSENCE OF SIMPLICITY .	15
III.	SIMPLICITY OF THOUGHT .	22
IV.	SIMPLICITY OF SPEECH . .	39
V.	SIMPLE DUTY	52
VI.	SIMPLE NEEDS	68
VII.	SIMPLE PLEASURES . . .	80
VIII.	THE MERCENARY SPIRIT AND SIMPLICITY	96
IX.	NOTORIETY AND THE INGLORIOUS GOOD	111

v

vi CONTENTS

PAGE

X. THE WORLD AND THE LIFE
OF THE HOME . . . 128

XI. SIMPLE BEAUTY 139

XII. PRIDE AND SIMPLICITY IN THE
INTERCOURSE OF MEN . . 151

XIII. THE EDUCATION FOR SIM-
PLICITY 167

XIV. CONCLUSION 188

THE SIMPLE LIFE

I

OUR COMPLEX LIFE

AT the home of the Blanchards, everything is topsy-turvy, and with reason. Think of it! Mlle. Yvonne is to be married Tuesday, and to-day is Friday! Callers loaded with gifts, and tradesmen bending under packages, come and go in endless procession. The servants are at the end of their endurance. As for the family and the betrothed, they no longer have a life or a fixed abode. Their mornings are spent with dressmakers, milliners, upholsterers, jewelers, decorators, and caterers. After that, comes a rush through offices, where one waits in line, gazing vaguely at busy clerks engulfed in papers. A fortunate thing, if there be time when this is over, to run home and dress for the series of ceremonial dinners — betrothal dinners, dinners of presentation, the settlement dinner, receptions, balls. About midnight, home again, harassed and weary, to find the latest accumulation of parcels, and a deluge of letters —

2   THE SIMPLE LIFE

congratulations, felicitations, acceptances and regrets
from bridesmaids and ushers, excuses of tardy tradesmen. And the *contretemps* of the last minute —
a sudden death that disarranges the bridal party ;
a wretched cold that prevents a favorite cantatrice
from singing, and so forth, and so forth. Those
poor Blanchards! They will never be ready, and
they thought they had foreseen everything!

Such has been their existence for a month. No
longer possible to breathe, to rest a half-hour, to
tranquillize one's thoughts. *No, this is not living!*

Mercifully, there is Grandmother's room. Grandmother is verging on eighty. Through many toils
and much suffering, she has come to meet things
with the calm assurance which life brings to men
and women of high thinking and large heart. She
sits there in her arm-chair, enjoying the silence of
long meditative hours. So the flood of affairs surg-
ing through the house, ebbs at her door. At the
threshold of this retreat, voices are hushed and
footfalls softened ; and when the young *fiancés*
want to hide away for a moment, they flee to
Grandmother.

"Poor children!" is her greeting. "You are
worn out! Rest a little and belong to each other.

OUR COMPLEX LIFE 3

All these things count for nothing. Don't let them absorb you, it isn't worth while."

They know it well, these two young people. How many times in the last weeks has their love had to make way for all sorts of conventions and futilities! Fate, at this decisive moment of their lives, seems bent upon drawing their minds away from the one thing essential, to harry them with a host of trivialities ; and heartily do they approve the opinion of Grandmamma when she says, between a smile and a caress :

" Decidedly, my dears, the world is growing too complex ; and it does not make people happier — quite the contrary !"

I ALSO, am of Grandmamma's opinion. From the cradle to the grave, in his needs as in his pleasures, in his conception of the world and of himself, the man of modern times struggles through a maze of endless complication. Nothing is simple any longer : neither thought nor action ; not pleasure, not even dying. With our own hands we have added to existence a train of hardships, and lopped off many a gratification. I believe that thousands of our fellow-men, suffering the consequences of a too

4 THE SIMPLE LIFE

artificial life, will be grateful if we try to give expression to their discontent, and to justify the regret for naturalness which vaguely oppresses them.

Let us first speak of a series of facts that put into relief the truth we wish to show.

The complexity of our life appears in the number of our material needs. It is a fact universally conceded, that our needs have grown with our resources. This is not an evil in itself; for the birth of certain needs is often a mark of progress. To feel the necessity of bathing, of wearing fresh linen, inhabiting wholesome houses, eating healthful food, and cultivating our minds, is a sign of superiority. But if certain needs exist by right, and are desirable, there are others whose effects are fatal, which, like parasites, live at our expense: numerous and imperious, they engross us completely.

Could our fathers have foreseen that we should some day have at our disposal the means and forces we now use in sustaining and defending our material life, they would have predicted for us an increase of independence, and therefore of happiness, and a decrease in competition for worldly goods: they might even have thought that through the simplification of life thus made possible, a higher degree of morality

OUR COMPLEX LIFE 5

would be attained. None of these things has come to pass. Neither happiness, nor brotherly love, nor power for good has been increased. In the first place, do you think your fellow-citizens, taken as a whole, are more contented than their forefathers, and less anxious about the future? I do not ask if they should find reason to be so, but if they really are so. To see them live, it seems to me that a majority of them are discontented with their lot, and, above all, absorbed in material needs and beset with cares for the morrow. Never has the question of food and shelter been sharper or more absorbing than since we are better nourished, better clothed, and better housed than ever. He errs greatly who thinks that the query, "What shall we eat, and what shall we drink, and wherewithal shall we be clothed?" presents itself to the poor alone, exposed as they are to the anguish of morrows without bread or a roof. With them the question is natural, and yet it is with them that it presents itself most simply. You must go among those who are beginning to enjoy a little ease, to learn how greatly satisfaction in what ·one has, may be disturbed by regret for what one lacks. And if you would see anxious care for future material good, material good in all its luxurious de-

THE SIMPLE LIFE

velopment, observe people of small fortune, and, above all, the rich. It is not the woman with one dress who asks most insistently how she shall be clothed, nor is it those reduced to the strictly necessary who make most question of what they shall eat to-morrow. As an inevitable consequence of the law that needs are increased by their satisfaction, *the more goods a man has, the more he wants.* The more assured he is of the morrow, according to the common acceptation, the more exclusively does he concern himself with how he shall live, and provide for his children and his children's children. Impossible to conceive of the fears of a man established in life — their number, their reach, and their shades of refinement.

From all this, there has arisen throughout the different social orders, modified by conditions and varying in intensity, a common agitation — a very complex mental state, best compared to the petulance of a spoiled child, at once satisfied and discontented.

OUR COMPLEX LIFE 7

IF we have not become happier, neither have we grown more peaceful and fraternal. The more desires and needs a man has, the more occasion he finds for conflict with his fellow-men; and these conflicts are more bitter in proportion as their causes are less just. It is the law of nature to fight for bread, for the necessities. This law may seem brutal, but there is an excuse in its very harshness, and it is generally limited to elemental cruelties. Quite different is the battle for the superfluous — for ambition, privilege, inclination, luxury. Never has hunger driven man to such baseness as have envy, avarice, and thirst for pleasure. Egotism grows more maleficent as it becomes more refined. We of these times have seen an increase of hostile feeling among brothers, and our hearts are less at peace than ever.*

After this, is there any need to ask if we have become better? Do not the very sinews of virtue lie in man's capacity to care for something outside himself? And what place remains for one's neighbor in a life given over to material cares, to artificial

---

* The author refers to the unparalleled bitterness of the conflict in France between Dreyfusards and anti-Dreyfusards.

8   THE SIMPLE LIFE

needs, to the satisfaction of ambitions, grudges, and whims? The man who gives himself up entirely to the service of his appetites, makes them grow and multiply so well that they become stronger than he; and once their slave, he loses his moral sense, loses his energy, and becomes incapable of discerning and practicing the good. He has surrendered himself to the inner anarchy of desire, which in the end gives birth to outer anarchy. In the moral life we govern ourselves. In the immoral life we are governed by our needs and passions; thus, little by little, the bases of the moral life shift, and the law of judgment deviates.

For the man enslaved to numerous and exacting needs, possession is the supreme good and the source of all other good things. It is true that in the fierce struggle for possession, we come to hate those who possess, and to deny the right of property when this right is in the hands of others and not in our own. But the bitterness of attack against others' possessions is only a new proof of the extraordinary importance we attach to possession itself. In the end, people and things come to be estimated at their selling price, or according to the profit to be drawn from them. What brings nothing is worth nothing;

OUR COMPLEX LIFE

he who has nothing, is nothing. Honest poverty risks passing for shame, and lucre, however filthy, is not greatly put to it to be accounted for merit.

Some one objects: "Then you make wholesale condemnation of progress, and would lead us back to the good old times — to asceticism perhaps."

Not at all. The desire to resuscitate the past is the most unfruitful and dangerous of Utopian dreams, and the art of good living does not consist in retiring from life. But we are trying to throw light upon one of the errors that drag most heavily upon human progress, in order to find a remedy for it — namely, the belief that man becomes happier and better by the increase of outward well-being. Nothing is falser than this pretended social axiom; on the contrary, that material prosperity without an offset, diminishes the capacity for happiness and debases character, is a fact which a thousand examples are at hand to prove. The worth of a civilization is the worth of the man at its center. When this man lacks moral rectitude, progress only makes bad worse, and further embroils social problems

10   THE SIMPLE LIFE

THIS principle may be verified in other domains than that of material well-being. We shall speak only of education and liberty. We remember when prophets in good repute announced that to transform this wicked world into an abode fit for the gods, all that was needed was the overthrow of tyranny, ignorance, and want—those three dread powers so long in league. To-day, other preachers proclaim the same gospel. We have seen that the unquestionable diminution of want has made man neither better nor happier. Has this desirable result been more nearly attained through the great care bestowed upon instruction? It does not yet appear so, and this failure is the despair of our national educators.

Then shall we stop the people's ears, suppress public instruction, close the schools? By no means. But education, like the mass of our age's inventions, is after all only a tool; everything depends upon the workman who uses it. . . . So it is with liberty. It is fatal or lifegiving according to the use made of it. Is it liberty still, when it is the prerogative of criminals or heedless blunderers? Liberty is an atmosphere of the higher life, and it is only by a slow and patient inward

OUR COMPLEX LIFE 11

transformation that one becomes capable of breathing it.

All life must have its law, the life of man so much the more than that of inferior beings, in that it is more precious and of nicer adjustment. This law for man is in the first place an external law, but it may become an internal law. When man has once recognized the inner law, and bowed before it, through this reverence and voluntary submission he is ripe for liberty: so long as there is no vigorous and sovereign inner law, he is incapable of breathing its air; for he will be drunken with it, maddened, morally slain. The man who guides his life by inner law, can no more live servile to outward authority than can the full-grown bird live imprisoned in the eggshell. But the man who has not yet attained to governing himself can no more live under the law of liberty than can the unfledged bird live without its protective covering. These things are terribly simple, and the series of demonstrations old and new that proves them, increases daily under our eyes. And yet we are as far as ever from understanding even the elements of this most important law. In our democracy, how many are there, great and small, who know, from having

12 THE SIMPLE LIFE

personally verified it, lived it and obeyed it, this truth without which a people is incapable of governing itself? Liberty? — it is respect; liberty? — it is obedience to the inner law; and this law is neither the good pleasure of the mighty, nor the caprice of the crowd, but the high and impersonal rule before which those who govern are the first to bow the head. Shall liberty, then, be proscribed? No; but men must be made capable and worthy of it, otherwise public life becomes impossible, and the nation, undisciplined and unrestrained, goes on through license into the inextricable tangles of demagoguery.

WHEN one passes in review the individual causes that disturb and complicate our social life, by whatever names they are designated, and their list would be long, they all lead back to one general cause, which is this: *the confusion of the secondary with the essential.* Material comfort, education, liberty, the whole of civilization — these things constitute the frame of the picture; but the frame no more makes the picture than the frock the monk or the uniform the soldier. Here the picture is man, and man with his most intimate possessions — namely, his conscience, his character

OUR COMPLEX LIFE 13

and his will. And while we have been elaborating and garnishing the frame, we have forgotten, neglected, disfigured the picture. Thus are we loaded with external good, and miserable in spiritual life; we have in abundance that which, if must be, we can go without, and are infinitely poor in the one thing needful. And when the depth of our being is stirred, with its need of loving, aspiring, fulfilling its destiny, it feels the anguish of one buried alive — is smothered under the mass of secondary things that weigh it down and deprive it of light and air.

We must search out, set free, restore to honor the true life, assign things to their proper places, and remember that the center of human progress is moral growth. What is a good lamp? It is not the most elaborate, the finest wrought, that of the most precious metal. A good lamp is a lamp that gives good light. And so also we are men and citizens, not by reason of the number of our goods and the pleasures we procure for ourselves, not through our intellectual and artistic culture, nor because of the honors and independence we enjoy; but by virtue of the strength of our moral fibre. And this is not a truth of to-day but a truth of all times.

14 THE SIMPLE LIFE

At no epoch have the exterior conditions which man has made for himself by his industry or his knowledge, been able to exempt him from care for the state of his inner life. The face of the world alters around us, its intellectual and material factors vary; and no one can arrest these changes, whose suddenness is sometimes not short of perilous. But the important thing is that at the center of shifting circumstance man should remain man, live his life, make toward his goal. And whatever be his road, to make toward his goal, the traveler must not lose himself in crossways, nor hamper his movements with useless burdens. Let him heed well his direction and forces, and keep good faith ; and that he may the better devote himself to the essential — which is to progress — at whatever sacrifice, let him simplify his baggage.

II

THE ESSENCE OF SIMPLICITY

BEFORE considering the question of a practical return to the simplicity of which we dream, it will be necessary to define simplicity in its very essence. For in regard to it people commit the same error that we have just denounced, confounding the secondary with the essential, substance with form. They are tempted to believe that simplicity presents certain external characteristics by which it may be recognized, and in which it really consists. Simplicity and lowly station, plain dress, a modest dwelling, slender means, poverty — these things seem to go together. Nevertheless, this is not the case. Just now I passed three men on the street : the first in his carriage ; the others on foot, and one of them shoeless. The shoeless man does not necessarily lead the least complex life of the three. It may be, indeed, that he who rides in his carriage is sincere and unaffected, in spite of

16 THE SIMPLE LIFE

his position, and is not at all the slave of his wealth ; it may be also that the pedestrian in shoes neither envies him who rides nor despises him who goes unshod ; and lastly, it is possible that under his rags, his feet in the dust, the third man has a hatred of simplicity, of labor, of sobriety, and dreams only of idleness and pleasure. For among the least simple and straightforward of men must be reckoned professional beggars, knights of the road, parasites, and the whole tribe of the obsequious and envious, whose aspirations are summed up in this : to arrive at seizing a morsel — the biggest possible — of that prey which the fortunate of earth consume. And to this same category, little matter what their station in life, belong the profligate, the arrogant, the miserly, the weak, the crafty. Livery counts for nothing : we must see the heart. No class has the prerogative of simplicity ; no dress, however humble in appearance, is its unfailing badge. Its dwelling need not be a garret, a hut, the cell of the ascetic nor the lowliest fisherman's bark. Under all the forms in which life vests itself, in all social positions, at the top as at the bottom of the ladder, there are people who live simply, and others who do not. We do not mean by this that simplicity betrays

THE ESSENCE OF SIMPLICITY   17

itself in no visible signs, has not its own habits, its
distinguishing tastes and ways; but this outward
show, which may now and then be counterfeited,
must not be confounded with its essence and its deep
and wholly inward source. *Simplicity is a state of
mind.* It dwells in the main intention of our lives.
A man is simple when his chief care is the wish to be
what he ought to be, that is, honestly and naturally
human.   And this is neither so easy nor so impossible as one might think.   At bottom, it consists in
putting our acts and aspirations in accordance with
the law of our being, and consequently with the
Eternal Intention which willed that we should be at
all.   Let a flower be a flower, a swallow a swallow, a
rock a rock, and let a man be a man, and not a fox,
a hare, a hog, or a bird of prey : this is the sum of
the whole matter.

Here we are led to formulate the practical ideal of
man.   Everywhere in life we see certain quantities
of matter and energy associated for certain ends.
Substances more or less crude are thus transformed
and carried to a higher degree of organization.   It
is not otherwise with the life of man.   The human
ideal is to transform life into something more excellent than itself.   We may compare existence to raw

18   THE SIMPLE LIFE

material. What it is, matters less than what is made of it, as the value of a work of art lies in the flowering of the workman's skill. We bring into the world with us different gifts : one has received gold, another granite, a third marble, most of us wood or clay. Our task is to fashion these substances. Everyone knows that the most precious material may be spoiled, and he knows, too, that out of the least costly an immortal work may be shaped. Art is the realization of a permanent idea in an ephemeral form. True life is the realization of the higher virtues, — justice, love, truth, liberty, moral power, — in our daily activities, whatever they may be. And this life is possible in social conditions the most diverse, and with natural gifts the most unequal. It is not fortune or personal advantage, but our turning them to account, that constitutes the value of life. Fame adds no more than does length of days : quality is the thing.

Need we say that one does not rise to this point of view without a struggle ? The spirit of simplicity is not an inherited gift, but the result of a laborious conquest. Plain living, like high thinking, is simplification. We know that science is the handful of ultimate principles gathered out of the tufted

THE ESSENCE OF SIMPLICITY 19

mass of facts; but what gropings to discover them! Centuries of research are often condensed into a principle that a line may state. Here the moral life presents strong analogy with the scientific. It, too, begins in a certain confusion, makes trial of itself, seeks to understand itself, and often mistakes. But by dint of action, and exacting from himself strict account of his deeds, man arrives at a better knowledge of life. Its law appears to him, and the law is this: *Work out your mission.* He who applies himself to aught else than the realization of this end, loses in living the *raison d'être* of life. The egoist does so, the pleasure-seeker, the ambitious: he consumes existence as one eating the full corn in the blade, — he prevents it from bearing its fruit; his life is lost. Whoever, on the contrary, makes his life serve a good higher than itself, saves it in giving it. Moral precepts, which to a superficial view appear arbitrary, and seem made to spoil our zest for life, have really but one object — to preserve us from the evil of having lived in vain. That is why they are constantly leading us back into the same paths; that is why they all have the same meaning: *Do not waste your life,* make it bear fruit; learn how to give it, in order that it may not con-

THE SIMPLE LIFE

sume itself! Herein is summed up the experience
of humanity, and this experience, which each man
must remake for himself, is more precious in proportion as it costs more dear. Illumined by its
light, he makes a moral advance more and more
sure. Now he has his means of orientation, his internal norm to which he may lead everything back ;
and from the vacillating, confused, and complex being that he was, he becomes simple. By the ceaseless influence of this same law, which expands
within him, and is day by day verified in fact, his
opinions and habits become transformed.

Once captivated by the beauty and sublimity of
the true life, by what is sacred and pathetic in this
strife of humanity for truth, justice, and brotherly
love, his heart holds the fascination of it. Gradu-
ally everything subordinates itself to this powerful and persistent charm. The necessary hierarchy
of powers is organized within him : the essential
commands, the secondary obeys, and order is born
of simplicity. We may compare this organization of
the interior life to that of an army. An army is
strong by its discipline, and its discipline consists in
respect of the inferior for the superior, and the con-
centration of all its energies toward a single end :

THE ESSENCE OF SIMPLICITY 21

discipline once relaxed, the army suffers. It will not do to let the corporal command the general. Examine carefully your life and the lives of others. Whenever something halts or jars, and complications and disorder follow, it is because the corporal has issued orders to the general. Where the natural law rules in the heart, disorder vanishes.

I despair of ever describing simplicity in any worthy fashion. All the strength of the world and all its beauty, all true joy, everything that consoles, that feeds hope, or throws a ray of light along our dark paths, everything that makes us see across our poor lives a splendid goal and a boundless future, comes to us from people of simplicity, those who have made another object of their desires than the passing satisfaction of selfishness and vanity, and have understood that the art of living is to know how to give one's life.

III

SIMPLICITY OF THOUGHT

IT is not alone among the practical manifestations of our life that there is need of making a clearing: the domain of our ideas is in
the same case. Anarchy reigns in human
thought: we walk in the woods, without compass or
sun, lost among the brambles and briars of infinite
detail.

When once man has recognized the fact that he
has an aim, and that this aim is *to be a man,* he or-
ganizes his thought accordingly. Every mode of
thinking or judging which does not make him better and stronger, he rejects as dangerous.

And first of all he flees the too common contrari-
ety of amusing himself with his thought. Thought
is a tool, with its own proper function: it isn't a
toy. Let us take an example. Here is the studio
of a painter. The implements are all in place:
everything indicates that this assemblage of means
is arranged with view to an end. Throw the room

SIMPLICITY OF THOUGHT 23

open to apes. They will climb on the benches, swing from the cords, rig themselves in draperies, coif themselves with slippers, juggle with brushes, nibble the colors, and pierce the canvases to see what is behind the paint. I don't question their enjoyment; certainly they must find this kind of exercise extremely interesting. But an atelier is not made to let monkeys loose in. No more is thought a ground for acrobatic evolutions. A man worthy of the name, thinks as he is, as his tastes are : he goes about it with his whole heart, and not with that fitful and sterile curiosity which, under pretext of observing and noting everything, runs the risk of never experiencing a deep and true emotion or accomplishing a right deed.

Another habit in urgent need of correction, ordinary attendant on conventional life, is the mania for examining and analyzing one's self at every turn. I do not invite men to neglect introspection and the examination of conscience. The endeavor to understand one's own mental attitudes and motives of conduct is an essential element of good living. But quite other is this extreme vigilance, this incessant observation of one's life and thoughts, this dissecting of one's self, like a piece of mechanism.

THE SIMPLE LIFE

It is a waste of time, and goes wide of the mark. The man who, to prepare himself the better for walking, should begin by making a rigid anatomical examination of his means of locomotion, would risk dislocating something before he had taken a step. You have what you need to walk with, then forward! Take care not to fall, and use your forces with discretion. Potterers and scruple-mongers are soon reduced to inaction. It needs but a glimmer of common sense to perceive that man is not made to pass his life in a self-centered trance.

And common sense — do you not find what is designated by this name becoming as rare as the common-sense customs of other days? Common sense has become an old story. We must have something new — and we create a factitious existence, a refinement of living, that the vulgar crowd has not the wherewithal to procure. It is so agreeable to be distinguished! Instead of conducting ourselves like rational beings, and using the means most obviously at our command, we arrive, by dint of absolute genius, at the most astonishing singularities. Better off the track than on the main line! All the bodily defects and deformities that orthopedy treats, give but a feeble idea of the

SIMPLICITY OF THOUGHT 25

humps, the tortuosities, the dislocations we have inflicted upon ourselves in order to depart from simple common sense; and at our own expense we learn that one does not deform himself with impunity. Novelty, after all, is ephemeral. Nothing endures but the eternal commonplace ; and if one departs from that, it is to run the most perilous risks. Happy he who is able to reclaim himself, who finds the way back to simplicity.

Good plain sense is not, as is often imagined, the innate possession of the first chance-comer, a mean and paltry equipment that has cost nothing to anyone. I would compare it to those old folk-songs, unfathered but deathless, which seem to have risen out of the very heart of the people. Good sense is a fund slowly and painfully accumulated by the labor of centuries. It is a jewel of the first water, whose value he alone understands who has lost it, or who observes the lives of others who have lost it. For my part, I think no price too great to pay for gaining it and keeping it, for the possession of eyes that see and a judgment that discerns. One takes good care of his sword, that it be not bent or rusted : with greater reason should he give heed to his thought.

26   THE SIMPLE LIFE

But let this be well understood : an appeal to common sense is not an appeal to thought that grovels, to narrow positivism which denies everything it cannot see or touch. For to wish that man should be absorbed in material sensations, to the exclusion of the high realities of the inner life, is also a want of good sense. Here we touch upon a tender point, round which the greatest battles of humanity are waging. In truth we are striving to attain a conception of life, searching it out amid countless obscurities and griefs: and everything that touches upon spiritual realities becomes day by day more painful. In the midst of the grave perplexities and transient disorders that accompany great crises of thought, it seems more difficult than ever to escape with any simple principles. Yet necessity itself comes to our aid, as it has done for the men of all times. The program of life is terribly simple, after all, and in the fact that existence so imperiously forces herself upon us, she gives us notice that she precedes any idea of her which we may make for ourselves, and that no one can put off living pending an attempt to understand life. Our philosophies, our explanations, our beliefs are everywhere confronted by facts, and these facts, prodi-

SIMPLICITY OF THOUGHT 27

gious, irrefutable, call us to order when we would
deduce life from our reasonings, and would wait
to act until we have ended philosophizing. It is
this happy necessity that prevents the world from
stopping while man questions his route. Travelers
of a day, we are carried along in a vast movement to
which we are called upon to contribute, but which
we have not foreseen, nor embraced in its entirety,
nor penetrated as to its ultimate aims. Our part is
to fill faithfully the rôle of private, which has de-
volved upon us, and our thought should adapt itself
to the situation. Do not say that we live in more
trying times than our ancestors, for things seen from
afar are often seen imperfectly: it is moreover
scarcely gracious to complain of not having been born
in the days of one's grandfather. What we may believe least contestable on the subject is this: from
the beginning of the world it has been hard to see
clearly; right thinking has been difficult everywhere and always. In the matter the ancients
were in no wise privileged above the moderns, and it
might be added that there is no difference between
men when they are considered from this point of
view. Master and servant, teacher and learner,
writer and artisan discern truth at the same cost.

28   THE SIMPLE LIFE

The light that humanity acquires in advancing is no
doubt of the greatest use ; but it also multiplies the
number and extent of human problems.   The difficulty is never removed, the mind always encounters
its obstacle.   The unknown controls us and hems us
in on all sides.   But just as one need not exhaust a
spring to quench his thirst, so we need not know
everything to live.   Humanity lives and always has
lived on certain elemental *provisions.*

We will try to point them out.   First of all, hu
manity lives by confidence.   In so doing it but
reflects, commensurate with its conscious thought,
that which is the hidden source of all beings.   An
imperturbable faith in the stability of the universe
and its intelligent ordering, sleeps in everything that
exists.   The flowers, the trees, the beasts of the
field, live in calm strength, in entire security.
There is confidence in the falling rain, in dawn-
ing day, in the brook running to the sea.   Everything that is seems to say : "I am, therefore I
should be ; there are good reasons for this, rest
assured."

So, too, mankind lives by confidence.   From the
simple fact that he is, man has within him the sufficient reason for his being — a pledge of assurance.

SIMPLICITY OF THOUGHT   29

He reposes in the power which has willed that he should be. To safeguard this confidence, to see that nothing disconcerts it, to cultivate it, render it more personal, more evident—toward this should tend the first effort of our thought. All that augments confidence within us is good, for from confidence is born the life without haste, tranquil energy, calm action, the love of life and its fruitful labor. Deep-seated confidence is the mysterious spring that sets in motion the energy within us. It is our nutriment. By it man lives, much more than by the bread he eats. And so everything that shakes this confidence is evil—poison, not food.

Dangerous is every system of thought that attacks the very fact of life, declaring it to be an evil. Life has been too often wrongly estimated in this century. What wonder that the tree withers when its roots are watered with corrosives. And there is an extremely simple reflection that might be made in the face of all this negation. You say life is an evil. Well; what remedy for it do you offer? Can you combat it, suppress it? I do not ask you to suppress your own life, to commit suicide;—of what advantage would that be to us?—but to suppress *life*, not merely human life, but life at its deep and hid-

30   THE SIMPLE LIFE

den origin, all this upspringing of existence **that**
pushes toward the light and, to your mind, is rushing to misfortune ; I ask you to suppress the will to
live that trembles through the immensities of space,
to suppress in short the source of life.   Can you do
it ? No.   Then leave us in peace.   Since no one
can hold life in check, is it not better to respect it
and use it than to go about making other people
disgusted with it ?   When one knows that certain
food is dangerous to health, he does not eat it, and
when a certain fashion of thinking robs us of confidence, cheerfulness and strength, we should reject
that, certain not only that it is a nutriment noxious
to the mind, but also that it is false.   There is no
truth for man but in thoughts that are human, and
pessimism is inhuman.   Besides, it wants as much in
modesty as in logic.   To permit one's self to count
as evil this prodigious thing that we call life, one
needs have seen its very foundation, almost to have
made it.   What a strange attitude is that of certain
great thinkers of our times ! They act as if they
had created the world, very long ago, in their youth,
but decidedly it was a mistake, and they had well
repented it.

Let us nourish ourselves from other meat;

SIMPLICITY OF THOUGHT 31

strengthen our souls with cheering thoughts. What
is truest for man is what best fortifies him.

IF mankind lives by confidence, it lives also by
hope — that form of confidence which turns
toward the future. All life is a result and an
aspiration, all that exists supposes an origin and tends
toward an end. Life is progression : progression is
aspiration. The progress of the future is an infini-
tude of hope. Hope is at the root of things, and
must be reflected in the heart of man. No hope, no
life. The same power which brought us into being,
urges us to go up higher. What is the meaning of
this persistent instinct which pushes us on? The
true meaning is that something is to result from life,
that out of it is being wrought a good greater than
itself, toward which it slowly moves, and that this
painful sower called man, needs, like every sower, to
count on the morrow. The history of humanity is
the history of indomitable hope ; otherwise everything would have been over long ago. To press
forward under his burdens, to guide himself in the
night, to retrieve his falls and his failures, to escape
despair even in death, man has need of hoping always, and sometimes against all hope. Here is the

32   THE SIMPLE LIFE

cordial that sustains him. Had we only logic, we
should have long ago drawn the conclusion : Death
has everywhere the last word ! — and we should be
dead of the idea. But we have hope, and that is
why we live and believe in life.

Suso, the great monk and mystic, one of the simplest and best men that ever lived, had a touching
custom : whenever he encountered a woman, were
she the poorest and oldest, he stepped respectfully
aside, though his bare feet must tread among thorns
or in the gutter. " I do that," he said, " to render
homage to our Holy Lady, the Virgin Mary." Let
us offer to hope a like reverence. If we meet it in
the shape of a blade of wheat piercing the furrow ;
a bird brooding on its nest ; a poor wounded beast,
recovering itself, rising and continuing its way ; a
peasant ploughing and sowing a field that has been
ravaged by flood or hail ; a nation slowly repairing
its losses and healing its wounds - — under whatever
guise of humanity or suffering it appears to us, let us
salute it ! When we encounter it in legends, in un-
tutored songs, in simple creeds, let us still salute it !
for it is always the same, indestructible, the immortal daughter of God.

We do not dare hope enough. The men of our

SIMPLICITY OF THOUGHT 35

day have developed strange timidities. The apprehension that the sky will fall — that acme of absurdity among the fears of our Gallic forefathers — has entered our own hearts. Does the rain-drop doubt the ocean? the ray mistrust the sun ? Our senile wisdom has arrived at this prodigy. It resembles those testy old pedagogues whose chief office is to rail at the merry pranks or the youthful enthusiasms of their pupils. It is time to become little children once more, to learn again to stand with clasped hands and wide eyes before the mystery around us ; to remember that, in spite of our knowledge, what we know is but a trifle, and that the world is greater than our mind, which is well ; for being so prodigious, it must hold in reserve untold resources, and we may allow it some credit without accusing ourselves of improvidence. Let us not treat it as creditors do an insolvent debtor: we should fire its courage, relight the sacred flame of hope. Since the sun still rises, since earth puts forth her blossoms anew, since the bird builds its nest, and the mother smiles at her child, let us have the courage to be men, and commit the rest to Him who has numbered the stars. For my part, I would I might find glowing words to say to whomsoever has lost heart in these times of disillu-

34 THE SIMPLE LIFE

sion: Rouse your courage, hope on; he is sure of
being least deluded who has the daring to do that;
the most ingenuous hope is nearer truth than the
most rational despair.

ANOTHER source of light on the path of
human life is goodness. I am not of those
who believe in the natural perfection of
man, and teach that society corrupts him. On the
contrary, of all forms of evil, the one which most
dismays me is heredity. But I sometimes ask myself how it is that this effete and deadly virus of low
instincts, of vices inoculated in the blood, the
whole assemblage of disabilities imposed upon us by
the past—how all this has not got the better of us.
It must be because of something else. This other
thing is love.

Given the unknown brooding above our heads, our
limited intelligence, the grievous and contradictory
enigma of human destiny, falsehood, hatred, corruption, suffering, death — what can we think, what do?
To all these questions a sublime and mysterious voice
has answered: *Love your fellow-men*. Love must indeed be divine, like faith and hope, since she cannot
die when so many powers are arrayed against her.

SIMPLICITY OF THOUGHT 35

She has to combat the natural ferocity of what may be called the beast in man; she has to meet ruse, force, self-interest, above all, ingratitude. How is it that she passes pure and scathless in the midst of these dark enemies, like the prophet of the sacred legend among the roaring beasts? It is because her enemies are of the earth, and love is from above. Horns, teeth, claws, eyes full of murderous fire, are powerless against the swift wing that soars toward the heights and eludes them. Thus love escapes the undertakings of her foes. She does even better: she has sometimes known the fine triumph of winning over her persecutors: she has seen the wild beasts grow calm, lie down at her feet, obey her law.

At the very heart of the Christian faith, the most sublime of its teachings, and to him who penetrates its deepest sense, the most human, is this: To save lost humanity, the invisible God came to dwell among us, in the form of a man, and willed to make Himself known by this single sign: *Love*.

Healing, consoling, tender to the unfortunate, even to the evil, love engenders light beneath her feet. She clarifies, she simplifies. She has chosen the humblest part — to bind up wounds, wipe away

36   THE SIMPLE LIFE

tears, relieve distress, soothe aching hearts, pardon, make peace; yet it is of love that we have the greatest need. And as we meditate on the best way to render thought fruitful, simple, really conformable to our destiny, the method sums itself up in these words: *Have confidence and hope; be kind.*

I would not discourage lofty speculation, dissuade any one whomsoever from brooding over the problems of the unknown, over the vast abysses of science or philosophy. But we have always to come back from these far journeys to the point where we are, often to a place where we seem to stand marking time with no result. There are conditions of life and social complications in which the sage, the thinker, and the ignorant are alike unable to see clearly. The present age has often brought us face to face with such situations; I am sure that he who meets them with our method will soon recognize its worth.

SINCE I have touched here upon religious ground, at least in a general way, someone may ask me to say in a few simple words, what religion is the best; and I gladly express myself on this subject. But it might be better not to

SIMPLICITY OF THOUGHT 37

put the question in this form. All religions have, of necessity, certain fixed characteristics, and each has its inherent qualities or defects. Strictly speaking, then, they may be compared among themselves: but there are always involuntary partialities or foregone conclusions. It is better to put the question otherwise, and ask: Is my own religion good, and how may I know it? To this question, this answer: Your religion is good if it is vital and active, if it nourishes in you confidence, hope, love, and a sentiment of the infinite value of existence; if it is allied with what is best in you against what is worst, and holds forever before you the necessity of becoming a new man; if it makes you understand that pain is a deliverer; if it increases your respect for the conscience of others; if it renders forgiveness more easy, fortune less arrogant, duty more dear, the beyond less visionary. If it does these things it is good, little matter its name: however rudimentary it may be, when it fills this office it comes from the true source, it binds you to man and to God.

But does it perchance serve to make you think yourself better than others, quibble over texts, wear sour looks, domineer over other's consciences or give your own over to bondage; stifle your scruples, fol-

38 THE SIMPLE LIFE

low religious forms for fashion or gain, do good in the hope of escaping future punishment ? — oh, then, if you proclaim yourself the follower of Buddha, Moses, Mahomet, or even Christ, your religion is worthless — it separates you from God and man.

I have not perhaps the right to speak thus in my own name; but others have so spoken before me who are greater than I, and notably He who recounted to the questioning scribe the parable of the Good Samaritan. I intrench myself behind His authority.

IV

SIMPLICITY OF SPEECH

SPEECH is the chief revelation of the mind, the first visible form that it takes. As the thought, so the speech. To better one's life in the way of simplicity, one must set a watch on his lips and his pen. Let the word be as genuine as the thought, as artless, as valid: think justly, speak frankly.

All social relations have their roots in mutual trust, and this trust is maintained by each man's sincerity. Once sincerity diminishes, confidence is weakened, society suffers, apprehension is born. This is true in the province of both natural and spiritual interests. With people whom we distrust, it is as difficult to do business as to search for scientific truth, arrive at religious harmony, or attain to justice. When one must first question words and intentions, and start from the premise that everything said and written is meant to offer us illusion in place of truth, life becomes strangely

40   THE SIMPLE LIFE

complicated. This is the case to-day. There is so much craft, so much diplomacy, so much subtle legerdemain, that we all have no end of trouble to inform ourselves on the simplest subject and the one that most concerns us. Probably what I have just said would suffice to show my thought, and each one's experience might bring to its support an ample commentary with illustrations. But I am none the less moved to insist on this point, and to strengthen my position with examples.

Formerly the means of communication between men were considerably restricted. It was natural to suppose that in perfecting and multiplying avenues of information, a better understanding would be brought about. Nations would learn to love each other as they became acquainted; citizens of one country would feel themselves bound in closer brotherhood as more light was thrown on what concerned their common life. When printing was invented, the cry arose: *fiat lux!* and with better cause when the habit of reading and the taste for newspapers increased. Why should not men have reasoned thus : — "Two lights illumine better than one, and many better than two : the more periodicals and books there are, the better we shall know

SIMPLICITY OF SPEECH 41

what happens, and those who wish to write history after us will be right fortunate; their hands will be full of documents"? Nothing could have seemed more evident. Alas! this reasoning was based upon the nature and capacity of the instruments, without taking into account the human element, always the most important factor. And what has really come about is this: that cavilers, calumniators, and crooks — all gentlemen glib of tongue, who know better than any one else how to turn voice and pen to account — have taken the utmost advantage of these extended means for circulating thought, with the result that the men of our times have the greatest difficulty in the world to know the truth about their own age and their own affairs. For every newspaper that fosters good feeling and good understanding between nations, by trying to rightly inform its neighbors and to study them without reservations, how many spread defamation and distrust! What unnatural and dangerous currents of opinion set in motion! what false alarms and malicious interpretations of words and facts! And in domestic affairs we are not much better informed than in foreign. As to commercial, industrial, and agricultural interests, political parties and social tendencies, or the personality of

THE SIMPLE LIFE

public men, it is alike difficult to obtain a disinterested opinion. The more newspapers one reads, the less clearly he sees in these matters. There are days when after having read them all, and admitting that he takes them at their word, the reader finds himself obliged to draw this conclusion: — Unquestionably nothing but corruption can be found any longer—no men of integrity except a few journalists. But the last part of the conclusion falls in its turn. It appears that the chroniclers devour each other. The reader has under his eyes a spectacle somewhat like the cartoon entitled, "The Combat of the Serpents." After having gorged themselves with everything around them, the reptiles fall upon each other, and there remain upon the field of battle two tails.

And not the common people alone feel this embarrassment, but the cultivated also — almost everybody shares it. In politics, finance, business — even in science, art, literature and religion, there is everywhere disguise, trickery, wire-pulling; one truth for the public, another for the initiated. The result is that everybody is deceived. It is vain to be behind the scenes on one stage; a man cannot be there on them all, and the very people who deceive others with the most ability, are in turn deceived when

SIMPLICITY OF SPEECH 43

they need to count upon the sincerity of their neighbors.

The result of such practices is the degradation of human speech. It is degraded first in the eyes of those who manipulate it as a base instrument. No word is respected by sophists, casuists, and quibblers, men who are moved only by a rage for gaining their point, or who assume that their interests are alone worth considering. Their penalty is to be forced to judge others by the rule they follow themselves: *Say what profits and not what is true.* They can no longer take any one seriously—a sad state of mind for those who write or teach ! How lightly must one hold his readers and hearers to approach them in such an attitude ! To him who has preserved enough honesty, nothing is more repugnant than the careless irony of an acrobat of the tongue or pen, who tries to dupe honest and ingenuous men. On one side openness, sincerity, the desire to be enlightened ; on the other, chicanery making game of the public ! But he knows not, the liar, how far he is misleading himself. The capital on which he lives is confidence, and nothing equals the confidence of the people, unless it be their distrust when once they find themselves be-

44   THE SIMPLE LIFE

trayed. They may follow for a time the exploiters of their artlessness, but then their friendly humor turns to hate. Doors which stood wide open offer an impassable front of wood, and ears once attentive are deaf. And the pity is that they have closed not to the evil alone, but to the good. This is the crime of those who distort and degrade speech: they shake confidence generally. We consider as a calamity the debasement of the currency, the lowering of interest, the abolition of credit:—there is a misfortune greater than these: the loss of confidence, of that moral credit which honest people give one another, and which makes speech circulate like an authentic currency. Away with counterfeiters, speculators, rotten financiers, for they bring under suspicion even the coin of the realm. Away with the makers of counterfeit speech, for because of them there is no longer confidence in anyone or anything, and what they say and write is not worth a continental.

You see how urgent it is that each should guard his lips, chasten his pen, and aspire to simplicity of speech. No more perversion of sense, circumlocution, reticence, tergiversation! these things serve only to complicate and bewilder. Be men; speak the speech

SIMPLICITY OF SPEECH 45

of honor. An hour of plain-dealing does more for the salvation of the world than years of duplicity.

A WORD now about a national bias, to those who have a veneration for diction and style. Assuredly there can be no quarrel with the taste for grace and elegance of speech. I am of opinion that one cannot say too well what he has to say. But it does not follow that the things best said and best written are most studied. Words should serve the fact, and not substitute themselves for it and make it forgotten in its embellishment. The greatest things are those which gain the most by being said most simply, since thus they show themselves for what they are : you do not throw over them the veil, however transparent, of beautiful discourse, nor that shadow so fatal to truth, called the writer's vanity. Nothing so strong, nothing so persuasive, as simplicity ! There are sacred emotions, cruel griefs, splendid heroisms, passionate enthusiasms that a look, a movement, a cry interprets better than beautifully rounded periods. The most precious possessions of the heart of humanity manifest themselves most simply. To be convincing, a thing must be true, and certain truths are more evident when they

46   THE SIMPLE LIFE

come in the speech of ingenuousness, even weakness, than when they fall from lips too well trained, or are proclaimed with trumpets. And these rules are good for each of us in his every-day life. No one can imagine what profit would accrue to his moral life from the constant observation of this principle: Be sincere, moderate, simple in the expression of your feelings and opinions, in private and public alike; never pass beyond bounds, give out faithfully what is within you, and above all, watch. — that is the main thing.

For the danger in fine words is that they live from a life of their own. They are servants of distinction, that have kept their titles but no longer perform their functions — of which royal courts offer us example. You speak well, write well, and all is said. How many people content themselves with speaking, and believe that it exempts them from acting! And those who listen are content with having heard them. So it sometimes happens that a life may in the end be made up of a few well-turned speeches, a few fine books, and a few great plays. As for practicing what is so magisterially set forth, that is the last thing thought of. And if we pass from the world of talent to spheres which the medi-

SIMPLICITY OF SPEECH 47

ocre exploit, there, in a pell-mell of confusion, we
see those who think that we are in the world to talk
and hear others talk — the great and hopeless rout
of babblers, of everything that prates, bawls, and per-
orates and, after all, finds that there isn't talking
enough. They all forget that those who make the
least noise do the most work. An engine that expends all its steam in whistling, has nothing left with
which to turn wheels. Then let us cultivate silence,
All that we can save in noise we gain in power.

THESE reflections lead us to consider a
similar subject, also very worthy of attention : I mean what has been called " the
vice of the superlative." If we study the inhabitants of a country, we notice differences of tem-
perament, of which the language shows signs.
Here the people are calm and phlegmatic ; their
speech is jejune, lacks color. Elsewhere tempera-
ments are more evenly balanced ; one finds pre-
cision, the word exactly fitted to the thing. But
farther on — effect of the sun, the air, the wine perhaps — hot blood courses in the veins, tempers are
excitable, language is extravagant, and the simplest
things are said in the strongest terms.

48   THE SIMPLE LIFE

If the type of speech varies with climate, it differs also with epochs. Compare the language, written or spoken, of our own times with that of certain other periods of our history. Under the old *régime*, people spoke differently than at the time of the Revolution, and we have not the same language as the men of 1830, 1848, or the Second Empire. In general, language is now characterized by greater simplicity: we no longer wear perukes, we no longer write in lace frills: but there is one significant difference between us and almost all of our ancestors — and it is the source of our exaggerations — our nervousness. Upon over-excited nervous systems — and Heaven knows that to have nerves is no longer an aristocratic privilege! — words do not produce the same impression as under normal conditions. And quite as truly, simple language does not suffice the man of over-wrought sensibilities when he tries to express what he feels. In private life, in public, in books, on the stage, calm and temperate speech has given place to excess. The means that novelists and playwrights employ to galvanize the public mind and compel its attention, are to be found again, in their rudiments, in our most commonplace conversations, in our letter-writing, and above all in public

SIMPLICITY OF SPEECH 49

speaking. Our performances in language compared to those of a man well-balanced and serene, are what our hand-writing is compared to that of our fathers. The fault is laid to steel pens. If only the truth were acknowledged ! — Geese, then, could save us ! But the evil goes deeper ; it is in ourselves. We write like men possessed : the pen of our ancestors was more restful, more sure. Here we face one of the results of our modern life, so complicated and so terribly exhaustive of energy. It leaves us impatient, breathless, in perpetual trepidation. Our handwriting, like our speech, suffers thereby and betrays us. Let us go back from the effect to the cause, and understand well the warning it brings us !

What good can come from this habit of exaggerated speech ? False interpreters of our own impressions, we can not but warp the minds of our fellow-men as well as our own. Between people who exaggerate, good understanding ceases. Ruffled tempers, violent and useless disputes, hasty judgments devoid of all moderation, the utmost extravagance in education and social life — these things are the result of intemperance of speech.

50   THE SIMPLE LIFE

MAY I be permitted, in this appeal for simplicity of speech, to frame a wish whose fulfilment would have the happiest results ? I ask for simplicity in literature, not only as one of the best remedies for the dejection of our souls — *blasés*, jaded, weary of eccentricities — but also as a pledge and source of social union. I ask also for simplicity in art. Our art and our literature are reserved for the privileged few of education and fortune. But do not misunderstand me. I do not ask poets, novelists, and painters to descend from the heights and walk along the mountain-sides, finding their satisfaction in mediocrity; but, on the contrary, to mount higher. The truly popular is not that which appeals to a certain class of society ordinarily called the common people; the truly popular is what is common to all classes and unites them. The sources of inspiration from which perfect art springs are in the depths of the human heart, in the eternal realities of life before which all men are equal. And the sources of a popular language must be found in the small number of simple and vigorous forms which express elementary sensations, and draw the master lines of human destiny. In them are truth,

SIMPLICITY OF SPEECH   51

power, grandeur, immortality.   Is there not enough
in such an ideal to kindle the enthusiasm of youth,
which, sensible that the sacred flame of the beautiful
is burning within, feels pity, and to the disdainful
adage, *Odi profanum vulgus*, prefers this more hu-
mane saying, *Misereor super turbam*.   As for me, I
have no artistic authority, but from out the multitude where I live, I have the right to raise my cry
to those who have been given talents, and say to
them: Labor for men whom the world forgets, make
yourselves intelligible to the humble, so shall you
accomplish a work of emancipation and peace; so
shall you open again the springs whence those masters drew, whose works have defied the ages because
they knew how to clothe genius in simplicity.

V

SIMPLE DUTY

WHEN we talk to children on a subject that annoys them, they call our attention to some pigeon on the roof, giving food to its little one, or some coachman down in the street who is abusing his horse. Sometimes they even maliciously propose one of those alarming questions that put the minds of parents on the rack; all this to divert attention from the distressing topic. I fear that in the face of duty we are big children, and, when that is the theme, seek subterfuges to distract us.

The first sophism consists in asking ourselves if there is such a thing as duty in the abstract, or if this word does not cover one of the numerous illusions of our forefathers. For duty, in truth, supposes liberty, and the question of liberty leads us into metaphysics. How can we talk of liberty so long as this grave problem of free-will is not solved? Theoretically there is no objection to this; and if

SIMPLE DUTY 53

life were a theory, and we were here to work out a complete system of the universe, it would be absurd to concern ourselves with duty until we had clarified the subject of liberty, determined its conditions, fixed its limits.

But life is not a theory. In this question of practical morality, as in the others, life has preceded hypothesis, and there is no room to believe that she ever yields it place. This liberty—relative, I admit, like everything we are acquainted with, for that matter — this duty whose existence we question, is none the less the basis of all the judgments we pass upon ourselves and our fellow-men. We hold each other to a certain extent responsible for our deeds and exploits.

The most ardent theorist, once outside of his theory, scruples not a whit to approve or disapprove the acts of others, to take measures against his enemies, to appeal to the generosity and justice of those he would dissuade from an unworthy step. One can no more rid himself of the notion of moral obligation than of that of time or space; and as surely as we must resign ourselves to walking before we know how to define this space through which we move and this time that measures our movements,

54   THE SIMPLE LIFE

so surely must we submit to moral obligation before having put our finger on its deep-hidden roots. Moral law dominates man, whether he respects or defies it. See how it is in every-day life: each one is ready to cast his stone at him who neglects a plain duty, even if he allege that he has not yet arrived at philosophic certitude. Everybody will say to him, and with excellent reason : "Sir, we are men before everything. First play your part, do your duty as citizen, father, son; after that you shall return to the course of your meditations."

However, let us be well understood. We should not wish to turn anyone away from scrupulous research into the foundations of morality. No thought which leads men to concern themselves once more with these grave questions, could be useless or indifferent. We simply challenge the thinker to find a way to wait till he has unearthed these foundations, before he does an act of humanity, of honesty or dishonesty, of valor or cowardice. And most of all do we wish to formulate a reply for all the insincere who have never tried to philosophize, and for ourselves when we would offer our state of philosophic doubt in justification of our practical omissions. From the simple fact that we

SIMPLE DUTY 55

are men, before all theorizing, positive, or negative, about duty, we have the peremptory law to conduct ourselves like men. There is no getting out of it.

But he little knows the resources of the human heart, who counts on the effect of such a reply. It matters not that it is itself unanswerable; it cannot keep other questions from arising. The sum of our pretexts for evading duty is equal to the sum of the sands of the sea or the stars of heaven.

We take refuge, then, behind duty that is obscure, difficult, contradictory. And these are certainly words to call up painful memories. To be a man of duty and to question one's route, grope in the dark, feel one's self torn between the contrary solicitations of conflicting calls, or again, to face a duty gigantic, overwhelming, beyond our strength — what is harder! And such things happen. We would neither deny nor contest the tragedy in certain situations or the anguish of certain lives. And yet, duty rarely has to make itself plain across such conflicting circumstances, or to be struck out from the tortured mind like lightning from a storm-cloud. Such formidable shocks are exceptional. Well for us if we stand staunch when they come! But if no one is astonished that oaks are uprooted by the

56 THE SIMPLE LIFE

whirlwind, that a wayfarer stumbles at night on an unknown road, or that a soldier caught between two fires is vanquished, no more should he condemn without appeal those who have been worsted in almost superhuman moral conflicts. To succumb under the force of numbers or obstacles has never been counted a disgrace.

So my weapons are at the service of those who intrench themselves behind the impregnable rampart of duty ill-defined, complicated or contradictory. But it is not that which occupies me to-day; it is of plain, I had almost said easy duty, that I wish to speak.

WE have yearly three or four high feast days, and many ordinary ones: there are likewise some very great and dark combats to wage, but beside these is the multitude of plain and simple duties. Now, while in the great encounters our equipment is generally adequate, it is precisely in the little emergencies that we are found wanting. Without fear of being misled by a paradoxical form of thought, I affirm, then, that the essential thing is to fulfil our simple duties and exercise elementary justice. In general, those

SIMPLE DUTY 57

who lose their souls do so not because they fail to rise to difficult duty, but because they neglect to perform that which is simple. Let us illustrate this truth.

He who tries to penetrate into the humble under-world of society is not slow to discover great misery, physical and moral. And the closer he looks, the greater number of unfortunates does he discover, till in the end this assembly of the wretched appears to him like a great black world, in whose presence the individual and his means of relief are reduced to helplessness. It is true that he feels impelled to run to the succor of these unfortunates, but at the same time he asks himself, "What is the use?" The case is certainly heartrending. Some, in despair, end by doing nothing. They lack neither pity nor good intention, but these bear no fruit. They are wrong. Often a man has not the means to do good on a large scale, but that is not a reason for failing to do it at all. So many people absolve themselves from any action, on the ground that there is too much to do! They should be recalled to simple duty, and this duty in the case of which we speak is that each one, according to his resources, leisure and capacity, should create relations for himself among

58   THE SIMPLE LIFE

the world's disinherited. There are people who by the exercise of a little good-will have succeeded in enrolling themselves among the followers of ministers, and have ingratiated themselves with princes. Why should you not succeed in forming relations with the poor, and in making acquaintances among the workers who lack somewhat the necessities of life? When a few families are known, with their histories, their antecedents and their difficulties, you may be of the greatest use to them by acting the part of a brother, with the moral and material aid that is yours to give. It is true, you will have attacked only one little corner, but you will have done what you could, and perhaps have led another on to follow you. Instead of stopping at the knowledge that much wretchedness, hatred, disunion and vice exist in society, you will have introduced a little good among these evils. And by however slow degrees such kindness as yours is emulated, the good will sensibly increase and the evil diminish. Even were you to remain alone in this undertaking, you would have the assurance that in fulfilling the duty, plain as a child's, which offered itself, you were doing the only reasonable thing. If you have felt it so, you **have** found out one of the secrets of right living.

SIMPLE DUTY 59

In its dreams, man's ambition embraces vast limits, but it is rarely given us to achieve great things, and even then, a quick and sure success always rests on a groundwork of patient preparation. Fidelity in small things is at the base of every great achievement. We too often forget this, and yet no truth needs more to be kept in mind, particularly in the troubled eras of history and in the crises of individual life. In shipwreck a splintered beam, an oar, any scrap of wreckage, saves us. On the tumbling waves of life, when everything seems shattered to fragments, let us not forget that a single one of these poor bits may become our plank of safety. To despise the remnants is demoralization.

You are a ruined man, or you are stricken by a great bereavement, or again, you see the fruit of toilsome years perish before your eyes. You cannot rebuild your fortune, raise the dead, recover your lost toil, and in the face of the inevitable, your arms drop. Then you neglect to care for your person, to keep your house, to guide your children. All this is pardonable, and how easy to understand! But it is exceedingly dangerous. To fold one's hands and let things take their course, is to transform one evil into worse. You who think that you

60 THE SIMPLE LIFE

have nothing left to lose, will by that very thought lose what you have. Gather up the fragments that remain to you, and keep them with scrupulous care. In good time this little that is yours will be your consolation. The effort made will come to your relief, as the effort missed will turn against you. If nothing but a branch is left for you to cling to, cling to that branch; and if you stand alone in defense of a losing cause, do not throw down your arms to join the rout. After the deluge a few sur vivors repeopled the earth. The future sometimes rests in a single life as truly as life sometimes hangs by a thread. For strength, go to history and Nature. From the long travail of both you will learn that failure and fortune alike may come from the slightest cause, that it is not wise to neglect detail, and, above all, that we must know how to wait and to begin again.

In speaking of simple duty I cannot help thinking of military life, and the examples it offers to combatants in this great struggle. He would little understand his soldier's duty who, the army once beaten, should cease to brush his garments, polish his rifle, and observe discipline. " But what would be the use?" perhaps you ask. Are there not vari-

SIMPLE DUTY 61

ous fashions of being vanquished ? Is it an indifferent matter to add to defeat, discouragement, disorder, and demoralization ? No, it should never be forgotten that the least display of energy in these terrible moments is a sign of life and hope. At once everybody feels that all is not lost.

During the disastrous retreat of 1813–1814, in the heart of the winter, when it had become almost impossible to present any sort of appearance, a general, I know not who, one morning presented himself to Napoleon, in full dress and freshly shaven. Seeing him thus, in the midst of the general demoralization, as elaborately attired as if for parade, the Emperor said : *My general, you are a brave man !*

AGAIN, the plain duty is the near duty. A very common weakness keeps many people from finding what is near them interesting ; they see that only on its paltry side. The distant, on the contrary, draws and fascinates them. In this way a fabulous amount of good-will is wasted. People burn with ardor for humanity, for the public good, for righting distant wrongs ; they walk through life, their eyes fixed on marvelous sights along the horizon, treading meanwhile on the feet

62 THE SIMPLE LIFE

of passers-by, or jostling them without being aware of their existence.

Strange infirmity, that keeps us from seeing our fellows at our very doors! People widely read and far-travelled are often not acquainted with their fellow-citizens, great or small. Their lives depend upon the coöperation of a multitude of beings whose lot remains to them quite indifferent. Not those to whom they owe their knowledge and culture, not their rulers, nor those who serve them and supply their needs, have ever attracted their attention. That there is ingratitude or improvidence in not knowing one's workmen, one's servants, all those in short with whom one has indispensable social relations — this has never come into their minds. Others go much farther. To certain wives, their husbands are strangers, and conversely. There are parents who do not know their children: their development, their thoughts, the dangers they run, the hopes they cherish, are to them a closed book. Many children do not know their parents, have no suspicion of their difficulties and struggles, no conception of their aims. And I am not speaking of those piteously disordered homes where all the relations are false, but of honorable families. Only,

SIMPLE DUTY

all these people are greatly preoccupied : each has his outside interest that fills all his time. The distant duty — very attractive, I don't deny — claims them entirely, and they are not conscious of the duty near at hand. I fear they will have their trouble for their pains. Each person's base of operations is the field of his immediate duty. Neglect this field, and all you undertake at a distance is compromised. First, then, be of your own country, your own city, your own home, your own church, your own work-shop ; then, if you can, set out from this to go beyond it. That is the plain and natural order, and a man must fortify himself with very bad reasons to arrive at reversing it. At all events, the result of so strange a confusion of duties is that many people employ their time in all sorts of affairs except those in which we have a right to demand it. Each is occupied with something else than what concerns him, is absent from his post, ignores his trade. This is what complicates life. And it would be so simple for each one to be about his own matter.

64 THE SIMPLE LIFE

ANOTHER form of simple duty. When damage is done, who should repair it? He who did it. This is just, but it is only theory, and the consequence of following the theory would be the evil in force until the malefactors were found and had offset it. But suppose they are not found? or suppose they can not or will not make amends?

The rain falls on your head through a hole in the roof, or the wind blows in at a broken window. Will you wait to find the man who caused the mischief? You would certainly think that absurd. And yet such is often the practice. Children indignantly protest, "I didn't put it there, and I shall not take it away!" And most men reason after the same fashion. It is logic. But it is not the kind of logic that makes the world move forward.

On the contrary, what we must learn, and what life repeats to us daily, is that the injury done by one must be repaired by another. One tears down, another builds up ; one defaces, another restores ; one stirs up quarrels, another appeases them ; one makes tears to flow, another wipes them away ; one lives for evil-doing, another dies for the right. And in the workings of this grievous law lies salvation.

SIMPLE DUTY 65

This also is logic, but a logic of facts which makes the logic of theories pale. The conclusion of the matter is not doubtful ; a single-hearted man draws it thus : given the evil, the great thing is to make it good, and to set about it on the spot; well indeed if Messrs. the Malefactors will contribute to the reparation ; but experience warns us not to count too much on their aid.

BUT however simple duty may be, there is still need of strength to do it. In what does this strength consist, or where is it found ? One could scarcely tire of asking. Duty is for man an enemy and an intruder, so long as it appears as an appeal from without. When it comes in through the door, he leaves by the window ; when it blocks up the windows, he escapes by the roof. The more plainly we see it coming, the more surely we flee. It is like those police, representatives of public order and official justice, whom an adroit thief succeeds in evading. Alas ! the officer, though he finally collar the thief, can only conduct him to the station, not along the right road. Before man is able to accomplish his duty, he must fall into the hands of another power than that which

66 THE SIMPLE LIFE

says, " Do this, do that ; shun this, shun that, or else beware ! "

This is an interior power ; it is love. When a man hates his work, or goes about it with indifference, all the forces of earth cannot make him follow it with enthusiasm. But he who loves his office moves of himself ; not only is it needless to compel him, but it would be impossible to turn him aside. And this is true of everybody. The great thing is to have felt the sanctity and immortal beauty in our obscure destiny ; to have been led by a series of experiences to love this life for its griefs and its hopes, to love men for their weakness and their greatness, and to belong to humanity through the heart, the intelligence and the soul. Then an unknown power takes possession of us, as the wind of the sails of a ship, and bears us toward pity and justice. And yielding to its irresistible impulse, we say : *I cannot help it, something is there stronger than I.* In so saying, the men of all times and places have designated a power that is above humanity, but which may dwell in men's hearts. And everything truly lofty within us appears to us as a manifestation of this mystery beyond. Noble feelings, like great thoughts and deeds, are things of inspiration. When the tree

SIMPLE DUTY 67

buds and bears fruit, it is because it draws vital
forces from the soil, and receives light and warmth
from the sun. If a man, in his humble sphere, in
the midst of the ignorance and faults that are his
inevitably, consecrates himself sincerely to his task,
it is because he is in contact with the eternal source
of goodness. This central force manifests itself under a thousand forms. Sometimes it is indomitable
energy; sometimes winning tenderness; sometimes
the militant spirit that grasps and uproots the evil;
sometimes maternal solicitude, gathering to its arms
from the wayside where it was perishing, some
bruised and forgotten life; sometimes the humble
patience of long research. All that it touches bears
its seal, and the men it inspires know that through
it we live and have our being. To serve it is their
pleasure and reward. They are satisfied to be its
instruments, and they no longer look at the outward
glory of their office, well knowing that nothing is
great, nothing small, but that our life and our deeds
are only of worth because of the spirit which breathes
through them.

VI

SIMPLE NEEDS

WHEN we buy a bird of the fancier, the good man tells us briefly what is necessary for our new pensioner, and the whole thing — hygiene, food, and the rest — is comprehended in a dozen words. Likewise, to sum up the necessities of most men, a few concise lines would answer. Their régime is in general of supreme simplicity, and so long as they follow it, all is well with them, as with every obedient child of Mother Nature. Let them depart from it, complications arise, health fails, gayety vanishes. Only simple and natural living can keep a body in full vigor. Instead of remembering this basic principle, we fall into the strangest aberrations.

What material things does a man need to live under the best conditions? A healthful diet, simple clothing, a sanitary dwelling-place, air and exercise. I am not going to enter into hygienic details, com-

SIMPLE NEEDS 69

pose menus, or discuss model tenements and dress reform. My aim is to point out a direction and tell what advantage would come to each of us from ordering his life in a spirit of simplicity. To know that this spirit does not rule in our society we need but watch the lives of men of all classes. Ask different people, of very unlike surroundings, this question : What do you need to live ? You will see how they respond. Nothing is more instructive. For some aboriginals of the Parisian asphalt, there is no life possible outside a region bounded by certain boulevards. There one finds the respirable air, the illuminating light, normal heat, classic cookery, and, in moderation, so many other things without which it would not be worth the while to promenade this round ball.

On the various rungs of the bourgeois ladder people reply to the question, what is necessary to live ? by figures varying with the degree of their ambition or education : and by education is oftenest understood the outward customs of life, the style of house, dress, table — an education precisely skindeep. Upward from a certain income, fee, or salary, life becomes possible : below that it is impossible. We have seen men commit suicide because their

THE SIMPLE LIFE

means had fallen under a certain minimum. They preferred to disappear rather than retrench. Observe that this minimum, the cause of their despair, would have been sufficient for others of less exacting needs, and enviable to men whose tastes are modest.

On lofty mountains vegetation changes with the altitude. There is the region of ordinary flora, that of the forests, that of pastures, that of bare rocks and glaciers. Above a certain zone wheat is no longer found, but the vine still prospers. The oak ceases in the low regions, the pine flourishes at considerable heights. Human life, with its needs, reminds one of these phenomena of vegetation.

At a certain altitude of fortune the financier thrives, the club-man, the society woman, all those in short for whom the strictly necessary includes a certain number of domestics and equipages, as well as several town and country houses. Further on flourishes the rich upper middle class, with its own standards and life. In other regions we find men of ample, moderate, or small means, and very unlike exigencies. Then come the people — artisans, day-laborers, peasants, in short, the masses, who live dense and serried like the thick, sturdy growths on

SIMPLE NEEDS 71

the summits of the mountains, where the larger vegetation can no longer find nourishment. In all these different regions of society men live, and no matter in which particular regions they flourish, all are alike human beings, bearing the same mark. How strange that among fellows there should be such a prodigious difference in requirements! And here the analogies of our comparison fail us. Plants and animals of the same families have identical wants. In human life we observe quite the contrary. What conclusion shall we draw from this, if not that with us there is a considerable elasticity in the nature and number of needs?

Is it well, is it favorable to the development of the individual and his happiness, and to the development and happiness of society, that man should have a multitude of needs, and bend his energies to their satisfaction? Let us return for a moment to our comparison with inferior beings. Provided that their essential wants are satisfied, they live content. Is this true of men? No. In all classes of society we find discontent. I leave completely out of the question those who lack the necessities of life. One cannot with justice count in the number of malcontents those from whom hunger, cold, and misery

72　THE SIMPLE LIFE

wring complaints. I am considering now that multitude of people who live under conditions at least supportable. Whence comes their heart-burning? Why is it found not only among those of modest though sufficient means, but also under shades of ever-increasing refinement, all along the ascending scale, even to opulence and the summits of social place? They talk of the contented middle classes. Who talk of them? People who, judging from without, think that as soon as one begins to enjoy ease he ought to be satisfied. But the middle classes themselves — do they consider themselves satisfied? Not the least in the world. If there are people at once rich and content, be assured that they are content because they know how to be so, not because they are rich. An animal is satisfied when it has eaten; it lies down and sleeps. A man also can lie down and sleep for a time, but it never lasts. When he becomes accustomed to this contentment, he tires of it and demands a greater. Man's appetite is not appeased by food; it increases with eating. This may seem absurd, but it is strictly true.

And the fact that those who make the most outcry are almost always those who should find the best reasons for contentment, proves unquestionably

SIMPLE NEEDS 73

that happiness is not allied to the number of our needs and the zeal we put into their cultivation. It is for everyone's interest to let this truth sink deep into his mind. If it does not, if he does not by decisive action succeed in limiting his needs, he risks a descent, insensible and beyond retreat, along the declivity of desire.

He who lives to eat, drink, sleep, dress, take his walk, — in short, pamper himself all that he can — be it the courtier basking in the sun, the drunken laborer, the commoner serving his belly, the woman absorbed in her toilettes, the profligate of low estate or high, or simply the ordinary pleasure-lover, a "good fellow," but too obedient to material needs — that man or woman is on the downward way of desire, and the descent is fatal. Those who follow it obey the same laws as a body on an inclined plane. Dupes of an illusion forever repeated, they think : " Just a few steps more, the last, toward the thing down there that we covet; then we will halt." But the velocity they gain sweeps them on, and the further they go the less able they are to resist it.

Here is the secret of the unrest, the madness, of many of our contemporaries. Having condemned their will to the service of their appetites, they

74 THE SIMPLE LIFE

suffer the penalty. They are delivered up to violent passions which devour their flesh, crush their bones, suck their blood, and cannot be sated. This is not a lofty moral denunciation. I have been listening to what life says, and have recorded, as I heard them, some of the truths that resound in every square.

Has drunkenness, inventive as it is of new drinks, found the means of quenching thirst? Not at all. It might rather be called the art of making thirst inextinguishable. Frank libertinage, does it deaden the sting of the senses? No; it envenoms it, converts natural desire into a morbid obsession and makes it the dominant passion. Let your needs rule you, pamper them — you will see them multiply like insects in the sun. The more you give them, the more they demand. He is senseless who seeks for happiness in material prosperity alone. As well undertake to fill the cask of the Danaïdes. To those who have millions, millions are wanting; to those who have thousands, thousands. Others lack a twenty-franc piece or a hundred sous. When they have a chicken in the pot, they ask for a goose; when they have the goose, they wish it were a turkey, and so on. We shall never learn how

SIMPLE NEEDS 75

fatal this tendency is. There are too many humble people who wish to imitate the great, too many poor working-men who ape the well-to-do middle classes, too many shop-girls who play at being ladies, too many clerks who act the club-man or sportsman; and among those in easy circumstances and the rich, are too many people who forget that what they possess could serve a better purpose than procuring pleasure for themselves, only to find in the end that one never has enough. Our needs, in place of the servants that they should be, have become a turbulent and seditious crowd, a legion of tyrants in miniature. A man enslaved to his needs may best be compared to a bear with a ring in its nose, that is led about and made to dance at will. The likeness is not flattering, but you will grant that it is true. It is in the train of their own needs that so many of those men are dragged along who rant for liberty, progress, and I don't know what else. They cannot take a step without asking them-selves if it might not irritate their masters. How many men and women have gone on and on, even to dishonesty, for the sole reason that they had too many needs and could not resign themselves to simple living! There are many guests in the cham-

76   THE SIMPLE LIFE

bers of Mazas who could give us much light on the
subject of too exigent needs.

Let me tell you the story of an excellent man
whom I knew.   He tenderly loved his wife and
children, and they all lived together, in France, in
comfort and plenty, but with little of the luxury
the wife coveted.   Always short of money, though
with a little management he might have been at
ease, he ended by exiling himself to a distant
colony, leaving his wife and children in the mother
country.   I don't know how the poor man can
feel off there ; but his family has a finer apartment,
more beautiful toilettes, and what passes for an
equipage.   At present they are perfectly contented,
but soon they will be used to this luxury — rudimentary after all.   Then Madam will find her furniture common and her equipage mean.   If this man
loves his wife — and that cannot be doubted — he
will migrate to the moon if there is hope of a larger
stipend.   In other cases the rôles are reversed, and
the wife and children are sacrificed to the ravenous
needs of the head of the family, whom an irregular
life, play, and countless other costly follies have
robbed of all dignity.   Between his appetites and
his rôle of father he has decided for the former,

SIMPLE NEEDS 77

and he slowly drifts toward the most abject egoism.

This forgetfulness of all responsibility, this gradual benumbing of noble feeling, is not alone to be found among pleasure-seekers of the upper classes : the people also are infected. I know more than one little household, which ought to be happy, where the mother has only pain and heartache day and night, the children are barefoot, and there is great ado for bread. Why? Because too much money is needed by the father. To speak only of the expenditure for alcohol, everybody knows the proportions that has reached in the last twenty years. The sums swallowed up in this gulf are fabulous — twice the indemnity of the war of 1870. How many legitimate needs could have been satisfied with that which has been thrown away on these artificial ones! The reign of wants is by no means the reign of brotherhood. The more things a man desires for himself, the less he can do for his neighbor, and even for those attached to him by ties of blood.

78 THE SIMPLE LIFE

THE destruction of happiness, independence, moral fineness, even of the sentiment of common interests — such is the result of the reign of needs. A multitude of other unfortunate things might be added, of which not the least is the disturbance of the public welfare. When society has too great needs, it is absorbed with the present, sacrifices to it the conquests of the past, immolates to it the future. After us the deluge! To raze the forests in order to get gold ; to squander your patrimony in youth, destroying in a day the fruit of long years ; to warm your house by burning your furniture ; to burden the future with debts for the sake of present pleasure; to live by expedients and sow for the morrow trouble, sickness, ruin, envy and hate — the enumeration of all the misdeeds of this fatal régime has no end.

On the other hand, if we hold to simple needs we avoid all these evils and replace them by measureless good. That temperance and sobriety are the best guardians of health is an old story. They spare him who observes them many a misery that saddens existence ; they insure him health, love of action, mental poise. Whether it be a question of food, dress, or dwelling, simplicity of taste is also a

SIMPLE NEEDS 79

source of independence and safety. The more simply you live, the more secure is your future; you are less at the mercy of surprises and reverses. An illness or a period of idleness does not suffice to dispossess you: a change of position, even considerable, does not put you to confusion. Having simple needs, you find it less painful to accustom yourself to the hazards of fortune. You remain a man, though you lose your office or your income, because the foundation on which your life rests is not your table, your cellar, your horses, your goods and chattels, or your money. In adversity you will not act like a nursling deprived of its bottle and rattle. Stronger, better armed for the struggle, presenting, like those with shaven heads, less advantage to the hands of your enemy, you will also be of more profit to your neighbor. For you will not rouse his jealousy, his base desires or his censure, by your luxury, your prodigality, or the spectacle of a sycophant's life; and, less absorbed in your own comfort, you will find the means of working for that of others.

VII

SIMPLE PLEASURES

DO you find life amusing in these days?
For my part, on the whole, it seems
rather depressing, and I fear that my
opinion is not altogether personal. As
I observe the lives of my contemporaries, and listen
to their talk, I find myself unhappily confirmed in
the opinion that they do not get much pleasure out
of things. And certainly it is not from lack of trying; but it must be acknowledged that their success
is meagre. Where can the fault be?

Some accuse politics or business; others social
problems or militarism. We meet only an embarrassment of choice when we start to unstring the
chaplet of our carking cares. Suppose we set out
in pursuit of pleasure. There is too much pep-
per in our soup to make it palatable. Our arms are
filled with a multitude of embarrassments, any one
of which would be enough to spoil our temper.
From morning till night, wherever we go, the people

SIMPLE PLEASURES 81

we meet are hurried, worried, preoccupied. Some have spilt their good blood in the miserable conflicts of petty politics : others are disheartened by the meanness and jealousy they have encountered in the world of literature or art. Commercial competition troubles the sleep of not a few. The crowded curricula of study and the exigencies of their opening careers, spoil life for young men. The working classes suffer the consequences of a ceaseless industrial struggle. It is becoming disagreeable to govern, because authority is diminishing ; to teach, because respect is vanishing. Wherever one turns there is matter for discontent.

And yet history shows us certain epochs of upheaval which were as lacking in idyllic tranquillity as is our own, but which the gravest events did not prevent from being gay. It even seems as if the seriousness of affairs, the uncertainty of the morrow, the violence of social convulsions, sometimes became a new source of vitality. It is not a rare thing to hear soldiers singing between two battles, and I think myself nowise mistaken in saying that human joy has celebrated its finest triumphs under the greatest tests of endurance. But to sleep peacefully on the eve of battle or to exult at the stake, men had

THE SIMPLE LIFE

then the stimulus of an internal harmony which we perhaps lack. Joy is not in things, it is in us, and I hold to the belief that the causes of our present unrest, of this contagious discontent spreading everywhere, are in us at least as much as in exterior conditions.

To give one's self up heartily to diversion one must feel himself on a solid basis, must believe in life and find it within him. And here lies our weakness. So many of us — even, alas! the younger men — are at variance with life ; and I do not speak of philosophers only. How do you think a man can be amused while he has his doubts whether after all life is worth living ? Besides this, one observes a disquieting depression of vital force, which must be attributed to the abuse man makes of his sensations. Excess of all kinds has blurred our senses and poisoned our faculty for happiness. Human nature succumbs under the irregularities imposed upon it. Deeply attainted at its root, the desire to live, persistent in spite of everything, seeks satisfaction in cheats and baubles. In medical science we have recourse to artificial respiration, artificial alimentation, and galvanism. So, too, around expiring pleasure we see a crowd of its votaries, ex-

SIMPLE PLEASURES 83

erting themselves to reawaken it, to reanimate it.
Most ingenious means have been invented ; it can
never be said that expense has been spared. Everything has been tried, the possible and the impossible. But in all these complicated alembics no one
has ever arrived at distilling a drop of veritable joy.
We must not confound pleasure with the instruments of pleasure. To be a painter, does it suffice
to arm one's self with a brush, or does the purchase
at great cost of a Stradivarius make one a musician ?
No more, if you had the whole paraphernalia of
amusement in the perfection of its ingenuity, would
it advance you upon your road. But with a bit of
crayon a great artist makes an immortal sketch.
It needs talent or genius to paint ; and to amuse
one's self, the faculty of being happy : whoever possesses it is amused at slight cost. This faculty is
destroyed by scepticism, artificial living, over-abuse ;
it is fostered by confidence, moderation and normal
habits of thought and action.

An excellent proof of my proposition, and one very
easily encountered, lies in the fact that wherever
life is simple and sane, true pleasure accompanies it
as fragrance does uncultivated flowers. Be this life
hard, hampered, devoid of all things ordinarily con-

84 THE SIMPLE LIFE

sidered as the very conditions of pleasure, the rare and delicate plant, joy, flourishes there. It springs up between the flags of the pavement, on an arid wall, in the fissure of a rock. We ask ourselves how it comes, and whence: but it lives; while in the soft warmth of conservatories or in fields richly fertilized you cultivate it at a golden cost to see it fade and die in your hand.

Ask actors what audience is happiest at the play; they will tell you the popular one. The reason is not hard to grasp. To these people the play is an exception, they are not bored by it from over-indulgence. And, too, to them it is a rest from rude toil. The pleasure they enjoy they have honestly earned, and they know its cost as they know that of each sou earned by the sweat of their labor. More, they have not frequented the wings, they have no intrigues with the actresses, they do not see the wires pulled. To them it is all real. And so they feel pleasure unalloyed. I think I see the sated sceptic, whose monocle glistens in that box, cast a disdainful glance over the smiling crowd.

"Poor stupid creatures, ignorant and gross!"

And yet they are the true livers, while he is an artificial product, a mannikin, incapable of experi-

SIMPLE PLEASURES 85

encing this fine and salutary intoxication **of an hour** of frank pleasure.

Unhappily, ingenuousness is disappearing, even in the rural districts. We see the people of our cities, and those of the country in **their turn, break-** ing with the good traditions. The mind, warped by alcohol, by the passion for gambling, and by unhealthy literature, contracts little by little perverted tastes. Artificial life makes irruption into communities once simple in their pleasures, and it is like phylloxera to the vine. The robust tree of rustic joy finds its sap drained, its leaves turning yellow.

Compare a *fête champêtre* of the good old style with the village festivals, so-called, of to-day. In the one case, in the honored setting of antique costumes, genuine countrymen sing the folk songs, dance rustic dances, regale themselves with native drinks, and seem entirely in their element. They take their pleasure as the blacksmith forges, as the cascade tumbles over the rocks, as the colts frisk in the meadows. It is contagious: it stirs your heart. In spite of yourself you are ready to cry: " Bravo, my children. That is fine ! " You want to join in. In the other case, you see villagers disguised as city folk, countrywomen made hideous

86 THE SIMPLE LIFE

by the modiste, and, as the chief ornament of the festival, a lot of degenerates who bawl the songs of music halls; and sometimes in the place of honor, a group of tenth-rate barnstormers, imported for the occasion, to civilize these rustics and give them a taste of refined pleasures. For drinks, liquors mixed with brandy or absinthe: in the whole thing neither originality nor picturesqueness. License, indeed, and clownishness, but not that *abandon* which ingenuous joy brings in its train.

THIS question of pleasure is capital. Staid people generally neglect it as a frivolity; utilitarians, as a costly superfluity. Those whom we designate as pleasure-seekers forage in this delicate domain like wild boars in a garden. No one seems to doubt the immense human interest attached to joy. It is a sacred flame that must be fed, and that throws a splendid radiance over life. He who takes pains to foster it accomplishes a work as profitable for humanity as he who builds bridges, pierces tunnels, or cultivates the ground. So to order one's life as to keep, amid toils and suffering, the faculty of happiness, and be able to propagate it in a sort of salutary contagion among one's

SIMPLE PLEASURES 87

fellow-men, is to do a work of fraternity in the
noblest sense. To give a trifling pleasure, smooth
an anxious brow, bring a little light into dark paths
— what a truly divine office in the midst of this
poor humanity ! But it is only in great simplicity
of heart that one succeeds in filling it.

We are not simple enough to be happy and to
render others so. We lack the singleness of heart
and the self-forgetfulness. We spread joy, as we
do consolation, by such methods as to obtain negative results. To console a person, what do we do ?
We set to work to dispute his suffering, persuade
him that he is mistaken in thinking himself
unhappy. In reality, our language translated into
truthful speech would amount to this : "You suffer, my friend ? That is strange ; you must be mistaken, for I feel nothing." As the only human
means of soothing grief is to share it in the heart,
how must a sufferer feel, consoled in this fashion ?

To divert our neighbor, make him pass an agreeable hour, we set out in the same way. We invite
him to admire our versatility, to laugh at our wit, to
frequent our house, to sit at our table ; through it
all, our desire to shine breaks forth. Sometimes,
also, with a patron's prodigality, we offer him the

88 THE SIMPLE LIFE

beneficence of a public entertainment of our own
choosing, unless we ask him to find amusement at
our home, as we sometimes do to make up a party
at cards, with the *arrière-pensée* of exploiting him to
our own profit. Do you think it the height of
pleasure for others to admire us, to admit our
superiority, and to act as our tools ? Is there anything in the world so disgusting as to feel one's self
patronized, made capital of, enrolled in a claque ?
To give pleasure to others and take it ourselves, we
have to begin by removing the ego, which is hateful, and then keep it in chains as long as the diver-
sions last. There is no worse kill-joy than the ego.
We must be good children, sweet and kind, button
our coats over our medals and titles, and with our
whole heart put ourselves at the disposal of others.

Let us sometimes live — be it only for an hour,
and though we must lay all else aside — to make
others smile. The sacrifice is only in appearance ;
no one finds more pleasure for himself than he who
knows how, without ostentation, to give himself
that he may procure for those around him a moment
of forgetfulness and happiness.

When shall we be so simply and truly *men* as not
to obtrude our personal business and distresses upon

SIMPLE PLEASURES 89

the people we meet socially? May we not forget for an hour our pretensions, our strife, our distributions into sets and cliques — in short, our "parts," and become as children once more, to laugh again that good laugh which does so much to make the world better?

HERE I feel drawn to speak of something very particular, and in so doing to offer my well-disposed readers an opportunity to go about a splendid business. I want to call their attention to several classes of people seldom thought of with reference to their pleasures.

It is understood that a broom serves only to sweep, a watering-pot to water plants, a coffee-mill to grind coffee, and likewise it is supposed that a nurse is designed only to care for the sick, a professor to teach, a priest to preach, bury, and confess, a sentinel to mount guard; and the conclusion is drawn that the people given up to the more serious business of life are dedicated to labor, like the ox. Amusement is incompatible with their activities. Pushing this view still further, we think ourselves warranted in believing that the infirm, the afflicted, the bankrupt, the vanquished in life's battle, and all

90 THE SIMPLE LIFE

those who carry heavy burdens, are in the shade, like the northern slopes of mountains, and that it is so of necessity. Whence the conclusion that serious people have no need of pleasure, and that to offer it to them would be unseemly; while as to the afflicted, there would be a lack of delicacy in breaking the thread of their sad meditations. It seems therefore to be understood that certain persons are condemned to be *always* serious, that we should approach them in a serious frame of mind, and talk to them only of serious things : so, too, when we visit the sick or unfortunate; we should leave our smiles at the door, compose our face and manner to dolefulness, and talk of anything heartrending. Thus we carry darkness to those in darkness, shade to those in shade. We increase the isolation of solitary lives and the monotony of the dull and sad. We wall up some existences as it were in dungeons ; and because the grass grows round their deserted prison-house, we speak low in approaching it, as though it were a tomb. Who suspects the work of infernal cruelty which is thus accomplished every day in the world ! This ought not to be.

When you find men or women whose lives are lost in hard tasks, or in the painful office of seeking

SIMPLE PLEASURES 91

out human wretchedness and binding up wounds, remember that they are beings made like you, that they have the same wants, that there are hours when they need pleasure and diversion. You will not turn them aside from their mission by making them laugh occasionally — these people who see so many tears and griefs; on the contrary, you will give them strength to go on the better with their work.

And when people whom you know are in trial, do not draw a sanitary cordon round them — as though they had the plague — that you cross only with precautions which recall to them their sad lot. On the contrary, after showing all your sympathy, all your respect for their grief, comfort them, help them to take up life again; carry them a breath from the out-of-doors — something in short to remind them that their misfortune does not shut them off from the world.

And so extend your sympathy to those whose work quite absorbs them, who are, so to put it, tied down. The world is full of men and women sacrificed to others, who never have either rest or pleasure, and to whom the least relaxation, the slightest respite, is a priceless good. And this minimum of

92 THE SIMPLE LIFE

comfort could be so easily found for them if only we thought of it. But the broom, you know, is made for sweeping, and it seems as though it could not be fatigued. Let us rid ourselves of this criminal blindness which prevents us from seeing the exhaustion of those who are always in the breach. Relieve the sentinels perishing at their posts, give Sisyphus an hour to breathe ; take for a moment the place of the mother, a slave to the cares of her house and her children ; sacrifice an hour of our sleep for someone worn by long vigils with the sick. Young girl, tired sometimes perhaps of your walk with your governess, take the cook's apron, and give her the key to the fields. You will at once make others happy and be happy yourself. We go unconcernedly along beside our brothers who are bent under burdens we might take upon ourselves for a minute. And this short respite would suffice to soothe aches, revive the flame of joy in many a heart, and open up a wide place for brotherliness. How much better would one understand another if he knew how to put himself heartily in that other's place, and how much more pleasure there would be in life !

SIMPLE PLEASURES 93

I HAVE spoken too fully elsewhere of systematizing amusements for the young, to return to it here in detail.*   But I wish to say in substance what cannot be too often repeated : If you wish youth to be moral, do not neglect its pleasures, or leave to chance the task of providing them.   You will perhaps say that young people do not like to have their amusements submitted to regulations, and that besides, in our day, they are already over-spoiled and divert themselves only too much.   I shall reply, first, that one may suggest ideas, indicate directions, offer opportunities for amusement, without making any regulations whatever.   In the second place, I shall make you see that you deceive yourselves in thinking youth has too much diversion. Aside from amusements that are artificial, enervating and immoral, that blight life instead of making it bloom in splendor, there are very few left to-day. Abuse, that enemy of legitimate use, has so befouled the world, that it is becoming difficult to touch anything but what is unclean : whence watchfulness, warnings and endless prohibitions.   One can hardly stir without encountering something that resembles unhealthy pleasure.   Among young people of to-

* See "Youth," the chapter on "Joy."

94   THE SIMPLE LIFE

day, particularly the self-respecting, the dearth of amusements causes real suffering. One is not weaned from this generous wine without discomfort. Impossible to prolong this state of affairs without deepening the shadow round the heads of the younger generations. We must come to their aid. Our children are heirs of a joyless world. We bequeath them cares, hard questions, a life heavy with shackles and complexities. Let us at least make an effort to brighten the morning of their days. Let us interest ourselves in their sports, find them pleasure-grounds, open to them our hearts and our homes. Let us bring the family into our amusements. Let gayety cease to be a commodity of export. Let us call in our sons, whom our gloomy interiors send out into the street, and our daughters, moping in dismal solitude. Let us multiply anniversaries, family parties, and excursions. Let us raise good humor in our homes to the height of an institution. Let the schools, too, do their part. Let masters and students — school-boys and college-boys — meet together oftener for amusement. It will be so much the better for serious work. There is no such aid to understanding one's professor as to have laughed in his company ; and conversely, to be well understood

SIMPLE PLEASURES 95

a pupil must be met elsewhere than in class or examination.

And who will furnish the money? What a question! That is exactly the error. Pleasure and money: people take them for the two wings of the same bird! A gross illusion! Pleasure, like all other truly precious things in this world, cannot be bought or sold. If you wish to be amused, you must do your part toward it; that is the essential. There is no prohibition against opening your purse, if you can do it, and find it desirable. But I assure you it is not indispensable. Pleasure and simplicity are two old acquaintances. Entertain simply, meet your friends simply. If you come from work well done, are as amiable and genuine as possible toward your companions, and speak no evil of the absent, your success is sure.

VIII

THE MERCENARY SPIRIT AND SIMPLICITY

WE have in passing touched upon a certain wide-spread prejudice which attributes to money a magic power. Having come so near enchanted ground we will not retire in awe, but plant a firm foot here, persuaded of many truths that should be spoken. They are not new, but how they are forgotten!

I see no possible way of doing without money. The only thing that theorists or legislators who accuse it of all our ills have hitherto achieved, has been to change its name or form. But they have never been able to dispense with a symbol representative of the commercial value of things. One might as well wish to do away with written language as to do away with money. Nevertheless, this question of a circulating medium is very troublesome. It forms one of the chief elements of

THE MERCENARY SPIRIT 97

complication in our life. The economic difficulties amid which we still flounder, social conventionalities, and the entire organization of modern life, have carried gold to a rank so eminent that it is not astonishing to find the imagination of man attributing to it a sort of royalty. And it is on this side that we shall attack the problem.

The term money has for appendage that of merchandise. If there were no merchandise there would be no money; but as long as there is merchandise there will be money, little matter under what form. The source of all the abuses which centre around money lies in a lack of discrimination. People have confused under the term and idea of merchandise, things which have no relation with one another. They have attempted to give a venal value to things which neither could have it nor ought to. The idea of purchase and sale has invaded ground where it may justly be considered an enemy and a usurper. It is reasonable that wheat, potatoes, wine, fabrics, should be bought and sold, and it is perfectly natural that a man's labor procure him rights to life, and that there be put into his hands something whose value represents them; but here already the analogy ceases to be

98 THE SIMPLE LIFE

complete. A man's labor is not merchandise in the same sense as a sack of flour or a ton of coal. Into this labor enter elements which cannot be valued in money. In short, there are things which can in no wise be bought: sleep, for instance, knowledge of the future, talent. He who offers them for sale must be considered a fool or an impostor. And yet there are gentlemen who coin money by such traffic. They sell what does not belong to them, and their dupes pay fictitious values in veritable coin. So, too, there are dealers in pleasure, dealers in love, dealers in miracles, dealers in patriotism, and the title of merchant, so honorable when it represents a man selling that which is in truth a commodity of trade, becomes the worst of stigmas when there is question of the heart, of religion, of country.

Almost all men are agreed that to barter with one's sentiments, his honor, his cloth, his pen, or his note, is infamous. Unfortunately this idea, which suffers no contradiction as a theory, and which thus stated seems rather a commonplace than a high moral truth, has infinite trouble to make its way in practice. Traffic has invaded the world. The money-changers are established even in the sanctu-

THE MERCENARY SPIRIT 99

ary, and by sanctuary I do not mean religious things alone, but whatever mankind holds sacred and inviolable. It is not gold that complicates, corrupts, and debases life; it is our mercenary spirit.

The mercenary spirit resolves everything into a single question: *How much is that going to bring me?* and sums up everything in a single axiom: *With money you can procure anything.* Following these two principles of conduct, a society may descend to a degree of infamy impossible to describe or to imagine.

How much is it going to bring me? This question, so legitimate while it concerns those precautions which each ought to take to assure his subsistence by his labor, becomes pernicious as soon as it passes its limits and dominates the whole life. This is so true that it vitiates even the toil which gains our daily bread. I furnish paid labor; nothing could be better: but if to inspire me in this labor I have only the desire to get the pay, nothing could be worse. A man whose only motive for action is his wages, does a bad piece of work: what interests him is not the doing, it's the gold. If he can retrench in pains without lessening his gains, be assured that he will do it. Plowman, mason, factory

THE SIMPLE LIFE

laborer, he who loves not his work puts into it neither interest nor dignity — is, in short, a bad workman. It is not well to confide one's life to a doctor who is wholly engrossed in his fees, for the spring of his action is the desire to garnish his purse with the contents of yours. If it is for his interest that you should suffer longer, he is capable of fostering your malady instead of fortifying your strength. The instructor of children who cares for his work only so far as it brings him profit, is a sad teacher ; for his pay is indifferent, and his teaching more indifferent still. Of what value is the mercenary journalist? The day you write for the dollar, your prose is not worth the dollar you write for. The more elevated in kind is the object of human labor, the more the mercenary spirit, if it be present, makes this labor void and corrupts it. There are a thousand reasons to say that all toil merits its wage, that every man who devotes his energies to providing for his life should have his place in the sun, and that he who does nothing useful, does not gain his livelihood, in short, is only a parasite. But there is no greater social error than to make gain the sole motive of action. The best we put into our work — be that work done by

THE MERCENARY SPIRIT   101

strength of muscle, warmth of heart, or concentra-
tion of mind — is precisely that for which no one
can pay us. Nothing better proves that man is not
a machine than this fact : two men at work with
the same forces and the same movements, produce
totally different results. Where lies the cause of
this phenomenon ? In the divergence of their
intentions. One has the mercenary spirit, the
other has singleness of purpose. Both receive
their pay, but the labor of the one is barren ; the
other has put his soul into his work. The work of
the first is like a grain of sand, out of which nothing
comes through all eternity ; the other's work is like
the living seed thrown into the ground ; it germinates and brings forth harvests. This is the secret
which explains why so many people have failed
while employing the very processes by which others
succeed. Automatons do not reproduce their kind,
and mercenary labor yields no fruit.

UNQUESTIONABLY we must bow before
economic facts, and recognize the difficulties of living : from day to day it becomes more imperative to combine well one's forces
in order to succeed in feeding, clothing, housing,

102 THE SIMPLE LIFE

and bringing up a family. He who does not rightly take account of these crying necessities, who makes no calculation, no provision for the future, is but a visionary or an incompetent, and runs the risk of sooner or later asking alms from those at whose parsimony he has sneered. And yet, what would become of us if these cares absorbed us entirely? if, mere accountants, we should wish to measure our effort by the money it brings, do nothing that does not end in a receipt, and consider as things worthless or pains lost whatever cannot be drawn up in figures on the pages of a ledger? Did our mothers look for pay in loving us and caring for us? What would become of filial piety if we asked it for loving and caring for our aged parents?

What does it cost you to speak the truth? Misunderstandings, sometimes sufferings and persecutions. To defend your country? Weariness, wounds and often death. To do good? Annoyance, ingratitude, even resentment. Self-sacrifice enters into all the essential actions of humanity. I defy the closest calculators to maintain their position in the world without ever appealing to aught but their calculations. True, those who know how to make their "pile" are rated as men of ability. But

THE MERCENARY SPIRIT   103

look a little closer.   How much of it do they owe to
the unselfishness of the simple-hearted?   Would
they have succeeded had they met only shrewd men
of their own sort, having for device: "No money
no service?"   Let us be outspoken; it is due to
certain people who do not count too rigorously, that
the world gets on.   The most beautiful acts of service and the hardest tasks have generally little re-
muneration or none.   Fortunately there are always
men ready for unselfish deeds; and even for those
paid only in suffering, though they cost gold, peace,
and even life.   The part these men play is often
painful and discouraging.   Who of us has not heard
recitals of experiences wherein the narrator regretted
some past kindness he had done, some trouble he
had taken, to have nothing but vexation in return?
These confidences generally end thus: "It was folly
to do the thing!"   Sometimes it is right so to
judge; for it is always a mistake to cast pearls before
swine; but how many lives there are whose sole acts
of real beauty are these very ones of which the doers
repent because of men's ingratitude!   Our wish for
humanity is that the number of these foolish deeds
may go on increasing.

104   THE SIMPLE LIFE

AND now I arrive at the *credo* of the mercenary spirit. It is characterized by brevity. For the mercenary man, the law and the prophets are contained in this one axiom : *With money you can get anything.* From a surface view of our social life, nothing seems more evident. " The sinews of war," " the shining mark," " the key that opens all doors," "king money!" — If one gathered up all the sayings about the glory and power of gold, he could make a litany longer than that which is chanted in honor of the Virgin. You must be without a penny, if only for a day or two, and try to live in this world of ours, to have any idea of the needs of him whose purse is empty. I invite those who love contrasts and unforeseen situations, to attempt to live without money three days, and far from their friends and acquaintances — in short, far from the society in which they are somebody. They will gain more experience in forty-eight hours than in a year otherwise. Alas for some people! they have this experience thrust upon them, and when veritable ruin descends around their heads, it is useless to remain in their own country, among the companions of their youth, their former colleagues, even those indebted to them. People affect to know them no

THE MERCENARY SPIRIT 105

longer. With what bitterness do they comment on the creed of money :—With gold one may have what he will ; without it, impossible to have anything ! They become pariahs, lepers, whom everyone shuns. Flies swarm round cadavers, men round gold. Take away the gold, nobody is there. Oh, it has caused tears to flow, this creed of gain ! bitter tears, tears of blood, even from those very eyes which once adored the golden calf.

And with it all, this creed is false, quite false. I shall not advance to the attack with hackneyed tales of the rich man astray in a desert, who cannot get even a drop of water for his gold ; or the decrepit millionaire who would give half he has to buy from a stalwart fellow without a cent, his twenty years and his lusty health. No more shall I attempt to prove that one cannot buy happiness. So many people who have money and so many more who have not would smile at this truth as the hardest ridden of saws. But I shall appeal to the common experience of each of you, to make you put your finger on the clumsy lie hidden beneath an axiom that all the world goes about repeating.

Fill your purse to the best of your means, and let us set out for one of the watering-places of which

106   THE SIMPLE LIFE

there are so many. I mean some little town formerly unknown and full of simple folk, respectful and hospitable, among whom it was good to be, and cost little. Fame with her hundred trumpets has announced them to the world, and shown them how they can profit from their situation, their climate, their personality. You start out, on the faith of Dame Rumor, flattering yourself that with your money you are going to find a quiet place to rest, and, far from the world of civilization and convention, weave a bit of poetry into the warp of your days.

The beginning is good. Nature's setting and some patriarchal costumes, slow to disappear, delight you. But as time passes, the impression is spoiled. The reverse side of things begins to show. This which you thought was as true antique as family heirlooms, is naught but trickery to mystify the credulous. Everything is labeled, all is for sale, from the earth to the inhabitants. These primitives have become the most consummate of sharpers. Given your money, they have resolved the problem of getting it with the least expense to themselves. On all sides are nets and traps, like spider-webs, and the fly that this gentry lies snugly

THE MERCENARY SPIRIT   107

in wait for is *you*. This is what twenty or thirty years of venality has done for a population once simple and honest, whose contact was grateful indeed to men worn by city life. Home-made bread has disappeared, butter comes from the dealer, they know to an art how to skim milk and adulterate wine ; they have all the vices of dwellers in cities without their virtues.

As you leave, you count your money. So much is wanting, that you make complaint. You are wrong. One never pays too dear for the conviction that there are things which money will not buy.

You have need in your house of an intelligent and competent servant: attempt to find this *rara avis*. According to the principle that with money one may get anything, you ought, as the position you offer is inferior, ordinary, good, or exceptional, to find servants unskilled, average, excellent, superior. But all those who present themselves for the vacant post are listed in the last category, and are fortified with certificates to support their pretensions. It is true that nine times out of ten, when put to the test, these experts are found totally wanting. Then why did they engage themselves with you ? They ought in truth to reply as does

108   THE SIMPLE LIFE

the cook in the comedy, who is dearly paid and proves to know nothing.

> "Why did you hire out as a *cordon bleu?*
> *It was to get bigger commissions.*"

That is the great affair. You will always find people who like to get big wages. More rarely you find capability. And if you are looking for probity, the difficulty increases. Mercenaries may be had for the asking; faithfulness is another thing. Far be it from me to deny the existence of faithful servants, at once intelligent and upright. But you will encounter as many, if not more, among the illy paid as among those most highly salaried. And it little matters where you find them, you may be sure that they are not faithful in their own interest; they are faithful because they have somewhat of that simplicity which renders us capable of self-abnegation.

We also hear on all sides the adage that money is the sinews of war. There is no question but that war costs much money, and we know something about it. Does this mean that in order to defend herself against her enemies and to honor her flag, a country need only be rich? In olden time the

THE MERCENARY SPIRIT 109

Greeks took it upon themselves to teach the Persians the contrary, and this lesson will never cease to be repeated in history. With money ships, cannon, horses may be bought; but not so military genius, administrative wisdom, discipline, enthusiasm. Put millions into the hands of your recruiters, and charge them to bring you a great leader and an army. You will find a hundred captains instead of one, and a thousand soldiers. But put them under fire: you will have enough of your hirelings! At least one might imagine that with money alone it is possible to lighten misery. Ah! that too is an illusion from which we must turn away. Money, be the sum great or small, is a seed which germinates into abuses. Unless there go with it intelligence, kindness, much knowledge of men, it will do nothing but harm, and we run great risk of corrupting both those who receive our bounty and those charged with its distribution.

MONEY will not answer for everything: it is a power, but it is not all-powerful. Nothing complicates life, demoralizes man, perverts the normal course of society like the development of venality. Wherever it reigns,

110   THE SIMPLE LIFE

everybody is duped by everybody else: one can no longer put trust in persons or things, no longer obtain anything of value.   We would not be detractors of money, but this general law must be applied to it: *Everything in its own place.*   When gold, which should be a servant, becomes a tyrannical power, affronting morality, dignity and liberty; when some exert themselves to obtain it at any price, offering for sale what is not merchandise, and others, possessing wealth, fancy that they can purchase what no one may buy, it is time to rise against this gross and criminal superstition, and cry aloud to the imposture: "Thy money perish with thee!" The most precious things that man possesses he has almost always received gratuitously: let him learn so to give them.

IX

NOTORIETY AND THE INGLORIOUS GOOD

ONE of the chief puerilities of our time is the love of advertisement. To emerge from obscurity, to be in the public eye, to make one's self talked of — some people are so consumed with this desire that we are justified in declaring them attacked with an itch for publicity. In their eyes obscurity is the height of ignominy : so they do their best to keep their names in every mouth. In their obscure position they look upon themselves as lost, like ship-wrecked sailors whom a night of tempest has cast on some lonely rock, and who have recourse to cries, volleys, fire, all the signals imaginable, to let it be known that they are there. Not content with setting off crackers and innocent rockets, many, to make themselves heard at any cost, have gone to the length of perfidy and even crime. The incendiary Erostratus has made numerous disciples. How many men of

112 THE SIMPLE LIFE

to-day have become notorious for having destroyed something of mark; pulled down — or tried to pull down — some man's high reputation; signalled their passage, in short, by a scandal, a meanness, or an atrocity!

This rage for notoriety does not surge through cracked brains alone, or only in the world of adventurers, charlatans and pretenders generally; it has spread abroad in all the domains of life, spiritual and material. Politics, literature, even science, and — most odious of all — philanthropy and religion are infected. Trumpets announce a good deed done, and souls must be saved with din and clamor. Pursuing its way of destruction, the rage for noise has entered places ordinarily silent, troubled spirits naturally serene, and vitiated in large measure all activity for good. The abuse of showing everything, or rather, putting everything on exhibition; the growing incapacity to appreciate that which chooses to remain hidden, and the habit of estimating the value of things by the racket they make, have come to corrupt the judgment of the most earnest men, and one sometimes wonders if society will not end by transforming itself into a great fair, with each one beating his drum in front of his tent.

NOTORIETY 113

Gladly do we quit the dust and din of like exhibitions, to go and breathe peacefully in some far-off nook of the woods, all surprise that the brook is so limpid, the forest so still, the solitude so enchanting. Thank God there are yet these uninvaded corners. However formidable the uproar, however deafening the babel of merry-andrews, it cannot carry beyond a certain limit; it grows faint and dies away. The realm of silence is vaster than the realm of noise. Herein is our consolation.

REST a moment on the threshold of this infinite world of inglorious good, of quiet activities. Instantly we are under the charm we feel in stretches of untrodden snow, in hiding wood-flowers, in disappearing pathways that seem to lead to horizons without bourn. The world is so made that the engines of labor, the most active agencies, are everywhere concealed. Nature affects a sort of coquetry in masking her operations. It costs you pains to spy her out, ingenuity to surprise her, if you would see anything but results and penetrate the secrets of her laboratories. Likewise in human society, the forces which move for good remain invisible, and even in our individual lives:

114 THE SIMPLE LIFE

what is best in us is incommunicable, buried in the depths of us. And the more vital are these sensibilities and intuitions, confounding themselves with the very source of our being, the less ostentatious they are: they think themselves profaned by exposure to the light of day. There is a secret and inexpressible joy in possessing at the heart of one's being, an interior world known only to God, whence, nevertheless, come impulses, enthusiasms, the daily renewal of courage, and the most powerful motives for activity among our fellow men. When this intimate life loses in intensity, when man neglects it for what is superficial, he forfeits in worth all that he gains in appearance. By a sad fatality, it happens that in this way we often become less admirable in proportion as we are more admired. And we remain convinced that what is best in the world is unknown there; for only those know it who possess it, and if they speak of it, in so doing they destroy its charm.

There are passionate lovers of nature whom she fascinates most in by-places, in the cool of forests, in the clefts of cañons, everywhere that the careless lover is not admitted to her contemplation. Forgetting time and the life of the world, they pass

NOTORIETY 115

days in these inviolate stillnesses, watching a bird build its nest or brood over its young, or some little groundling at its gracious play So to seek the good within himself — one must go where he no longer finds constraint, or pose, or "gallery" of any sort, but the simple fact of a life made up of wishing to be what it is good for it to be, without troubling about anything else,

May we be permitted to record here some obser‑ vations made from life ? As no names are given, they cannot be considered indiscreet.

In my country of Alsace, on the solitary route whose interminable ribbon stretches on and on under the forests of the Vosges, there is a stone‑ breaker whom I have seen at his work for thirty years. The first time I came upon him, I was a young student, setting out with swelling heart for the great city. The sight of this man did me good, for he was humming a song as he broke his stones. We exchanged a few words, and he said at the end : "Well, good-by, my boy, good courage and good luck!" Since then I have passed and repassed along that same route, under circumstances the most diverse, painful and joyful The student has finished his course, the breaker of stones

116 THE SIMPLE LIFE

remains what he was. He has taken a few more precautions against the seasons' storms: a rush-mat protects his back, and his felt hat is drawn further down to shield his face. But the forest is always sending back the echo of his valiant hammer. How many sudden tempests have broken over his bent back, how much adverse fate has fallen on his head, on his house, on his country ' He continues to break his stones, and, coming and going I find him by the roadside, smiling in spite of his age and his wrinkles, benevolent, speaking — above all in dark days — those simple words of brave men, which have so much effect when they are scanned to the breaking of stones.

It would be quite impossible to express the emotion the sight of this simple man gives me, and certainly he has no suspicion of it. I know of nothing more reassuring and at the same time more searching for the vanity which ferments in our hearts, than this coming face to face with an obscure worker who does his task as the oak grows and as the good God makes his sun to rise, without asking who is looking on.

I have known, too, a number of old teachers, men and women who have passed their whole life at the

NOTORIETY

same occupation — making the rudiments of human knowledge and a few principles of conduct penetrate heads sometimes harder than the rocks They have done it with their whole soul, throughout the length of a hard life in which the attention of men had little place. When they lie in their unknown graves, no one remembers them but a few humble people like themselves But their recompense is in their love. No one is greater than these unknown.

How many hidden virtues may one not discover — if he know how to search — among people of a class he often ridicules without perceiving that in so doing he is guilty of cruelty, ingratitude and stupidity : I mean old maids. People amuse themselves with remarking the surprising dress and ways of some of them — things of no consequence, for that matter. They persist also in reminding us that others, very selfish, take interest in nothing but their own comfort and that of some cat or canary upon which their powers of affection center ; and certainly these are not outdone in egoism by the most hardened celibates of the stronger sex. But what we oftenest forget is the amount of self-sacrifice hidden modestly away in so many of these truly admirable lives. Is it nothing to be without home and its love, with-

118   THE SIMPLE LIFE

out future, without personal ambition? to take upon
one's self that cross of solitary life, so hard to bear,
especially when there is added the solitude of the
heart? to forget one's self and have no other interests
than the care of the old, of orphans, the poor, the
infirm — those whom the brutal mechanism of life
casts out among its waste? Seen from without, these
apparently tame and lusterless lives rouse pity rather
than envy. Those who approach gently sometimes
divine sad secrets, great trials undergone, heavy
burdens beneath which too fragile shoulders bend;
but this is only the side of shadow. We should learn
to know and value this richness of heart, this pure
goodness, this power to love, to console, to hope, this
joyful giving up of self, this persistence in sweetness
and forgiveness even toward the unworthy. Poor
old maids! how many wrecked lives have you
rescued, how many wounded have you healed, how
many wanderers have you gently led aright, how
many naked have you clothed, how many orphans
have you taken in, and how many strangers, who
would have been alone in the world but for you —
you who yourselves are often remembered of no
one. I mistake. Someone knows you; it is that
great mysterious Pity which keeps watch over our

NOTORIETY 119

lives and suffers in our misfortunes. Forgotten like you, often blasphemed, it has confided to you some of its heavenliest messages, and that perhaps is why above your gentle comings and goings, we sometimes seem to hear the rustling wings of ministering angels.

THE good hides itself under so many different forms, that one has often as much pains to discover it as to unearth the best concealed crimes. A Russian doctor, who had passed ten years of his life in Siberia, condemned for political reasons to forced labor, used to find great pleasure in telling of the generosity, courage and humanity he had observed, not only among a large number of the condemned, but also among the convict guards. For the moment one is tempted to exclaim: Where will not the good hide away! And in truth life offers here great surprises and embarrassing contrasts. There are good men, officially so recognized, quoted among their associates, I had almost said guaranteed by the Government or the Church, who can be reproached with nothing but dry and hard hearts; while we are astonished to encounter in certain fallen human

120   THE SIMPLE LIFE

beings, the most genuine tenderness, and as it were a thirst for self-devotion.

I SHOULD like to speak next — apropos of the inglorious good — of a class that to-day it is thought quite fitting to treat with the utmost one-sidedness. I mean the rich. Some people think the last word is said when they have stigmatized that infamy, capital. For them, all who possess great fortunes are monsters gorged with the blood of the miserable. Others, not so declamatory, persist, however, in confounding riches with egoism and insensibility. Justice should be visited on these errors, be they involuntary or calculated. No doubt there are rich men who concern themselves with nobody else, and others who do good only with ostentation; indeed, we know it too well. But does their inhumanity or hypocrisy take away the value of the good that others do, and that they often hide with a modesty so perfect?

I knew a man to whom every misfortune had come which can strike us in our affections. He had lost a beloved wife, had seen all his children buried, one after another. But he had a great fortune, the result of his own labor. Living in the utmost sim

NOTORIETY 121

plicity, almost without personal wants, he spent his
time in searching for opportunities to do good, and
profiting by them. How many people he surprised
in flagrant poverty, what means he combined for re-
lieving distress and lighting up dark lives, with what
kindly thoughtfulness he took his friends unawares,
no one can imagine. He liked to do good to others
and enjoy their surprise when they did not know
whence the relief came. It pleased him to repair
the injustices of fortune, to bring tears of happiness
in families pursued by mischance. He was continually plotting, contriving, machinating in the dark,
with a childish fear of being caught with his hand
in the bag. The greater part of these fine deeds
were not known till after his death; the whole of
them we shall never know.

He was a socialist of the right sort! for there
are two kinds of them. Those who aspire to appro-
priate to themselves a part of the goods of others,
are numerous and commonplace. To belong to
their order it suffices to have a big appetite.
Those who are hungering to divide their own goods
with men who have none, are rare and precious, for
to enter this choice company there is need of a
brave and noble heart, free from selfishness, and

122   THE SIMPLE LIFE

sensitive to both the happiness and unhappiness of
its fellows.   Fortunately the race of these socialists
is not extinct, and I feel an unalloyed satisfaction in
offering them a tribute they never claim.

I must be pardoned for dwelling upon this.   It
does one good to offset the bitterness of so many in-
famies, so many calumnies, so much charlatanism, by
resting the eyes upon something more beautiful,
breathing the perfume of these stray corners where
simple goodness flowers.

A lady, a foreigner, doubtless little used to Parisian life, just now told me with what horror the
things she sees here inspire her : — these vile post-
ers, these "yellow" journals, these women with
bleached hair, this crowd rushing to the races, to
dance-halls, to roulette tables, to corruption — the
whole flood of superficial and mundane life.   She
did not speak the word Babylon, but doubtless it
was out of pity for one of the inhabitants of this
city of perdition.

"Alas, yes, madam, these things are sad, but you
have not seen all."

"Heaven preserve me from that!"

"On the contrary, I wish you could see everything; for if the dark side is very ugly, there is so

NOTORIETY 123

much to atone for it. And believe me, madam, you have simply to change your quarter, or observe at another hour. For instance, take the Paris of early morning. It will offer much to correct your impressions of the Paris of the night. Go see, among so many other working people, the street-sweepers, who come out at the hour when the revellers and malefactors go in. Observe beneath these rags those caryatid bodies, those austere faces! How serious they are at their work of sweeping away the refuse of the night's revelry. One might liken them to the prophets at Ahasuerus's gates. There are women among them, many old people. When the air is cold they stop to blow their fingers, and then go at it again. So it is every day. And they, too, are inhabitants of Paris.

Go next to the faubourgs, to the factories, especially the smaller ones, where the children or the employers labor with the men. Watch the army of workers marching to their tasks. How ready and willing these young girls seem, as they come gaily down from their distant quarters to the shops and stores and offices of the city. Then visit the homes from which they come. See the woman of the people at her work. Her husband's wages are modest,

124 THE SIMPLE LIFE

their dwelling is cramped, the children are many, the father is often harsh. Make a collection of the biographies of lowly people, budgets of modest family life: look at them attentively and long.

After that, go see the students. Those who have scandalized you in the streets are numerous, but those who labor hard are legion — only they stay at home, and are not talked about. If you knew the toil and dig of the Latin Quarter! You find the papers full of the rumpus made by a certain set of youths who call themselves students. The papers say enough of those who break windows; but why do they make no mention of those who spend their nights toiling over problems? Because it wouldn't interest the public. Yes, when now and then one of them, a medical student perhaps, dies a victim to professional duty, the matter has two lines in the dailies. A drunken brawl gets half a column, with every detail elaborated. Nothing is lacking but the portraits of the heroes — and not always that!

I should never end were I to try to point out to you all that you must go to see if you would see all: you would needs make the tour of society at large, rich and poor, wise and ignorant. And certainly you would not judge so severely then. Paris

NOTORIETY 125

is a world, and here, as in the world in general, the good hides away while the evil flaunts itself. Observing only the surface, you sometimes ask how there can possibly be so much riff-raff. When, on the contrary, you look into the depths, you are astonished that in this troublous, obscure and sometimes frightful life there can be so much of virtue.

BUT why linger over these things?. Am I not blowing trumpets for those who hold trumpet-blowing in horror? Do not understand me so. My aim is this — to make men think about unostentatious goodness; above all, to make them love it and practice it. The man who finds his satisfaction in things which glitter and hold his eyes, is lost: first, because he will thus see evil before all else; then, because he gets accustomed to the sight of only such good as seeks for notice, and therefore easily succumbs to the temptation to live himself for appearances. Not only must one be resigned to obscurity, he must love it, if he does not wish to slip insensibly into the ranks of figurants, who preserve their parts only while under the eyes of the spectators, and put off in the wings the restraints imposed on the stage.

126   THE SIMPLE LIFE

Here we are in the presence of one of the essential elements of the moral life. And this which we say is true not only for those who are called humble and whose lot it is to pass unremarked ; it is just as true, and more so, for the chief actors. If you would not be a brilliant inutility, a man of gold lace and plumes, but empty inside, you must play the star rôle in the simple spirit of the most obscure of your collaborators. He who is nothing worth except on hours of parade, is worth less than nothing. Have we the perilous honor of being always in view, of marching in the front ranks ? Let us take so much the greater care of the sanctuary of silent good within us. Let us give to the structure whose façade is seen of our fellowmen, a wide foundation of simplicity, of humble fidelity. And then, out of sympathy, out of gratitude, let us stay near our brothers who are unknown to fame. We owe everything to them — do we not ? I call to witness everyone who has found in life this encouraging experience, that stones hidden in the soil hold up the whole edifice. All those who arrive at having a public and recognized value, owe it to some humble spiritual ancestors, to some forgotten inspirers. A small number of the good, among them

NOTORIETY 127

simple women, peasants, vanquished heroes, parents
as modest as they are revered, personify for us
beautiful and noble living ; their example inspires
us and gives us strength. The remembrance of
them is forever inseparable from that conscience
before which we arraign ourselves. In our hours
of trial, we think of them, courageous and serene,
and our burdens lighten. In clouds they compass
us about, these witnesses invisible and beloved who
keep us from stumbling and our feet from falling
in the battle ; and day by day do they prove to us
that the treasure of humanity is its hidden goodness.

X

THE WORLD AND THE LIFE OF THE HOME

IN the time of the Second Empire, in one of our pleasantest sub-prefectures of the provinces, a little way from some baths frequented by the Emperor, there was a mayor, a very worthy man and intelligent too, whose head was suddenly turned by the thought that his sovereign might one day descend upon his home. Up to this time he had lived in the house of his fathers, a son respectful of the slightest family traditions. But when once the all-absorbing idea of receiving the Emperor had taken possession of his brain, he became another man. In this new light, what had before seemed sufficient for his needs, even enjoyable, all this simplicity that his ancestors had loved, appeared poor, ugly, ridiculous. Out of the question to ask an Emperor to climb this wooden staircase, sit in these old arm-chairs, walk over such superannuated carpets. So the mayor called architect

128

THE LIFE OF THE HOME 129

and masons ; pickaxes attacked walls and demolished partitions, and a drawing-room was made, out of all proportion to the rest of the house in size and splendor. He and his family retired into close quarters, where people and furniture incommoded each other generally. Then, having emptied his purse and upset his household by this stroke of genius, he awaited the royal guest. Alas, he soon saw the end of the Empire arrive, but the Emperor never.

The folly of this poor man is not so rare. As mad as he are all those who sacrifice their home life to the demands of the world. And the danger in such a sacrifice is most menacing in times of unrest. Our contemporaries are constantly exposed to it, and constantly succumbing. How many family treasures have they literally thrown away to satisfy worldly ambitions and conventions ; but the happiness upon which they thought to come through these impious immolations always eludes them.

To give up the ancestral hearth, to let the family traditions fall into desuetude, to abandon the simple domestic customs, for whatever return, is to make a fool's bargain ; and such is the place in society of family life, that if this be impoverished, the trouble

130   THE SIMPLE LIFE

is felt throughout the whole social organism. To
enjoy a normal development, this organism has need
of well-tried individuals, each having his own value,
his own hall-mark. Otherwise society becomes a
flock, and sometimes a flock without a shepherd.
But whence does the individual draw his originality
— this unique something, which, joined to the dis-
tinctive qualities of others, constitutes the wealth
and strength of a community? He can draw it only
from his own family. Destroy the assemblage of
memories and practices whence emanates for each
home an atmosphere in miniature, and you dry up
the sources of character, sap the strength of public
spirit.

It concerns the country that each home be a
world, profound, respected, communicating to its
members an ineffaceable moral imprint. But before
pursuing the subject further, let us rid ourselves of a
misunderstanding. Family feeling, like all beautiful
things, has its caricature, which is family egoism.
Some families are like barred and bolted citadels,
their members organized for the exploitation of the
whole world. Everything that does not directly
concern them is indifferent to them. They live like
colonists, I had almost said intruders, in the society

THE LIFE OF THE HOME   131

around them. Their particularism is pushed to such.
an excess that they make enemies of the whole human race. In their small way they resemble those
powerful societies, formed from time to time through
the ages, which possess themselves of universal rule,
and for which no one outside their own community
counts. This is the spirit that has sometimes made
the family seem a retreat of egoism which it was
necessary to destroy for the public safety. But as
patriotism and jingoism are as far apart as the east
from the west, so are family feeling and clannish-
ness.

HERE we are talking of right family feeling,
and nothing else in the world can take its
place; for in it lie in germ all those fine
and simple virtues which assure the strength and
duration of social institutions. And the very base of
family feeling is respect for the past; for the best
possessions of a family are its common memories.
An intangible, indivisible and inalienable capital,
these souvenirs constitute a sacred fund that each
member of a family ought to consider more precious
than anything else he possesses. They exist in a
dual form : in idea and in fact. They show them-

132   THE SIMPLE LIFE

selves in language, habits of thought, sentiments, even instincts, and one sees them materialized in portraits, furniture, buildings, dress, songs. To profane eyes, they are nothing ; to the eyes of those who know how to appreciate the things of the family, they are relics with which one should not part at any price.

But what generally happens in our day ? Worldliness wars upon the sentiment of family, and I know of no strife more impassioned. By great means and small, by all sorts of new customs, requirements and pretensions, the spirit of the world breaks into the domestic sanctuary. What are this stranger's rights? its titles? Upon what does it rest its peremptory claims ? This is what people too often neglect to inquire. They make a mistake. We treat the invader as very poor and simple people do a pompous visitor. For this incommoding guest of a day, they pillage their garden, bully their children and servants, and neglect their work. Such conduct is not only wrong, it is impolitic. One should have the courage to remain what he is, in the face of all comers.

The worldly spirit is full of impertinences. Here is a home which has formed characters of mark, and

THE LIFE OF THE HOME   133

is forming them yet. The people, the furnishings, the customs are all in harmony. By marriage or through relations of business or pleasure, the worldly spirit enters. It finds everything out of date, awkward, too simple, lacking the modern touch. At first it restricts itself to criticism and light raillery. But this is the dangerous moment. Look out for yourself; here is the enemy! If you so much as listen to his reasonings, to-morrow you will sacrifice a piece of furniture, the next day a good old tradition, and so one by one the family heirlooms dear to the heart will go to the bric-a-brac dealer — and filial piety with them.

In the midst of your new habits and in the changed atmosphere, your friends of other days, your old relatives, will be expatriated. Your next step will be to lay them aside in their turn; the worldly spirit leaves the old out of consideration. At last, established in an absolutely transformed setting, even you will view yourself with amazement. Nothing will be familiar, but surely it will be correct; at least the world will be satisfied! — Ah! that is where you are mistaken! After having made you cast out pure treasure as so much junk, it will find that your borrowed livery fits you ill, and

134   THE SIMPLE LIFE

will hasten to make you sensible of the ridiculous-ness of the situation.   Much better have had from the beginning the courage of your convictions, and have defended your home.

Many young people when they marry, listen to this voice of the world.   Their parents have given them the example of a modest life; but the new generation thinks it affirms its rights to existence and liberty, by repudiating ways in its eyes too patriarchal.   So these young folks make efforts to set themselves up lavishly in the latest fashion, and rid themselves of useless property at dirt-cheap prices.   Instead of filling their houses with objects which say: Remember! they garnish them with quite new furnishings that as yet have no meaning. Wait, I am wrong; these things are often symbols, as it were, of a facile and superficial existence.   In their midst one breathes a certain heady vapor of mundanity.   They recall the life outside, the tur-moil, the rush.   And were one sometimes disposed to forget this life, they would call back his wandering thought and say: Remember! — in another sense: Do not forget your appointment at the club, the play, the races!   The home, then, becomes a sort of half-way house where one comes to rest a little

THE LIFE OF THE HOME   135

between two prolonged absences ; it isn't a good place to stay. As it has no soul, it does not speak to yours. Time to eat and sleep, and then off again ! Otherwise you become as dull as a hermit.

We are all acquainted with people who have a rage for being abroad, who think the world would no longer go round if they didn't figure on all sides of it. To stay at home is penal ; there they cease to be in view. A horror of home life possesses them to such a degree that they would rather pay to be bored outside than be amused gratuitously within.

In this way society slowly gravitates toward life in herds, which must not be confounded with public life. The life in herds is somewhat like that of swarms of flies in the sun. Nothing so much resembles the worldly life of a man as the worldly life of another man. And this universal banality destroys the very essence of public spirit. One need not journey far to discover the ravages made in modern society by the spirit of worldliness ; and if we have so little foundation, so little equilibrium, calm good sense and initiative, one of the chief reasons lies in the undermining of the home life. The masses

136   THE SIMPLE LIFE

have timed their pace by that of people of fashion. They too have become worldly. Nothing can be more so than to quit one's own hearth for the life of saloons. The squalor and misery of the homes is not enough to explain the current which carries each man away from his own. Why does the peasant desert for the inn the house that his father and grandfather found so comfortable ? It has remained the same. There is the same fire in the same chimney. Whence comes it that it lights only an incomplete circle, when in olden times young and old sat shoulder to shoulder? Something has changed in the minds of men. Yielding to dangerous impulses, they have broken with simplicity. The fathers have quitted their post of honor, the wives grow dull beside the solitary hearth, and the children quarrel while waiting their turn to go abroad, each after his own fancy.

We must learn again to live the home life, to value our domestic traditions. A pious care has preserved certain monuments of the past. So antique dress, provincial dialects, old folk songs have found appreciative hands to gather them up before they should disappear from the earth. What a good deed, to guard these crumbs of a great past, these vestiges of the souls of our ancestors ! Let us

THE LIFE OF THE HOME   137

do the same for our family traditions, save and guard as much as possible of the patriarchal, whatever its form.

B UT not everyone has traditions to keep. All the more reason for redoubling the effort to constitute and foster a family life. And to do this there is need neither of numbers nor a rich establishment. To create a home you must have the spirit of home. Just as the smallest village may have its history, its moral stamp, so the smallest home may have its soul. Oh ! the spirit of places, the atmosphere which surrounds us in human dwellings ! What a world of mystery ! Here, even on the threshold the cold begins to penetrate, you are ill at ease, something intangible repulses you. There, no sooner does the door shut you in than friendliness and good humor envelop you. It is said that walls have ears. They have also voices, a mute eloquence. Everything that a dwelling contains is bathed in an ether of personality. And I find proof of its quality even in the apartments of bachelors and solitary women. What an abyss between one room and another room ! Here, all is dead, indifferent, common-

THE SIMPLE LIFE

place: the device of the owner is written all over it, even in his fashion of arranging his photographs and books: All is the same to me! There, one breathes in animation, a contagious joy in life. The visitor hears repeated in countless fashions: "Whoever you are, guest of an hour, I wish you well, peace be with you!"

Words can do little justice to the subject of home, tell little about the effect of a favorite flower in the window, or the charm of an old armchair where the grandfather used to sit, offering his wrinkled hands to the kisses of chubby children. Poor moderns, always moving or remodeling! We who from transforming our cities, our houses, our customs and creeds, have no longer where to lay our heads, let us not add to the pathos and emptiness of our changeful existence by abandoning the life of the home. Let us light again the flame put out on our hearths, make sanctuaries for ourselves, warm nests where the children may grow into men, where love may find privacy, old age repose, prayer an altar, and the fatherland a cult!

XI

SIMPLE BEAUTY

SOMEONE may protest against the nature of the simple life in the name of esthetics, or oppose to ours the theory of the service of luxury — that providence of business, fostering mother of arts, and grace of civilized society. We shall try, briefly, to anticipate these objections.

It will no doubt have been evident that the spirit which animates these pages is not utilitarian. It would be an error to suppose that the simplicity we seek has anything in common with that which misers impose upon themselves through cupidity, or narrow-minded people through false austerity. To the former the simple life is the one that costs least; to the latter it is a flat and colorless existence, whose merit lies in depriving one's self of everything bright, smiling, seductive.

It displeases us not a whit that people of large means should put their fortune into circulation instead of hoarding it, so giving life to commerce and

140 THE SIMPLE LIFE

the fine arts. That is using one's privileges to good advantage. What we would combat is foolish prodigality, the selfish use of wealth, and above all the quest of the superfluous on the part of those who have the greatest need of taking thought for the necessary. The lavishness of a Mæcenas could not have the same effect in a society as that of a common spendthrift who astonishes his contemporaries by the magnificence of his life and the folly of his waste. In these two cases the same term means very different things — to scatter money broadcast does not say it all; there are ways of doing it which ennoble men, and others which degrade them. Besides, to scatter money supposes that one is well provided with it. When the love of sumptuous living takes possession of those whose means are limited, the matter becomes strangely altered. And a very striking characteristic of our time is the rage for scattering broadcast which the very people have who ought to husband their resources. Munificence is a benefit to society, that we grant willingly. Let us even allow that the prodigality of certain rich men is a safety-valve for the escape of the superabundant: we shall not attempt to gainsay it. Our contention is that too many people meddle with the

SIMPLE BEAUTY 141

safety-valve when to practice economy is the part of both their interest and their duty : their extravagance is a private misfortune and a public danger.

SO much for the utility of luxury.

We now wish to explain ourselves upon the question of esthetics — oh ! very modestly, and without trespassing on the ground of the specialists. Through a too common illusion, simplicity and beauty are considered as rivals. But simple is not synonymous with ugly, any more than sumptuous, stylish and costly are synonymous with beautiful. Our eyes are wounded by the crying spectacle of gaudy ornament, venal art and senseless and graceless luxury. Wealth coupled with bad taste sometimes makes us regret that so much money is in circulation to provoke the creation of such a prodigality of horrors. Our contemporary art suffers as much from the want of simplicity as does our literature — too much in it that is irrelevant, overwrought, falsely imagined. Rarely is it given us to contemplate in line, form, or color, that simplicity allied to perfection which commands the eyes as evidence does the mind. We need to be rebaptized in the ideal purity of immortal beauty which puts its

142 THE SIMPLE LIFE

seal on the masterpieces; one shaft of its radiance
is worth more than all our pompous exhibitions.

YET what we now have most at heart is to
speak of the ordinary esthetics of life, of
the care one should bestow upon the adorn-
ment of his dwelling and his person, giving to existence that luster without which it lacks charm. For
it is not a matter of indifference whether man pays
attention to these superfluous necessities or whether
he does not: it is by them that we know whether
he puts soul into his work. Far from considering
it as wasteful to give time and thought to the perfecting, beautifying and poetizing of forms, I think
we should spend as much as we can upon it. Nature gives us her example, and the man who should
affect contempt for the ephemeral splendor of beauty
with which we garnish our brief days, would lose
sight of the intentions of Him who has put the
same care and love into the painting of the lily of
an hour and the eternal hills.

But we must not fall into the gross error of confounding true beauty with that which has only the
name. The beauty and poetry of existence lie in
the understanding we have of it. Our home, our

SIMPLE BEAUTY 143

table, our dress should be the interpreters of intentions. That these intentions be so expressed, it is first necessary to have them, and he who possesses them makes them evident through the simplest means. One need not be rich to give grace and charm to his habit and his habitation : it suffices to have good taste and good-will. We come here to a point very important to everybody, but perhaps of more interest to women than to men.

Those who would have women conceal themselves in coarse garments of the shapeless uniformity of bags, violate nature in her very heart, and misunderstand completely the spirit of things. If dress were only a precaution to shelter us from cold or rain, a piece of sacking or the skin of a beast would answer. But it is vastly more than this. Man puts himself entire into all that he does ; he transforms into types the things that serve him. The dress is not simply a covering, it is a symbol. I call to witness the rich flowering of national and provincial costumes, and those worn by our early corporations. A woman's toilette, too, has something to say to us. The more meaning there is in it, the greater its worth. To be truly beautiful, it must tell us of beautiful things, things personal and veritable.

144   THE SIMPLE LIFE

Spend all the money you possess upon it, if its form is determined by chance or custom, if it has no relation to her who wears it, it is only toggery, a domino. Ultra-fashionable dress, which completely masks feminine personality under designs of pure convention, despoils it of its principal attraction. From this abuse it comes about that many things which women admire do as much wrong to their beauty as to the purses of their husbands and fathers. What would you say of a young girl who expressed her thoughts in terms very choice, indeed, but taken word for word from a phrase-book? What charm could you find in this borrowed language? The effect of toilettes well-designed in themselves but seen again and again on all women indiscriminately, is precisely the same.

I can not resist citing here a passage from Camille Lemonnier, that harmonizes with my idea.

"Nature has given to the fingers of woman a charming art, which she knows by instinct, and which is peculiarly her own — as silk to the worm, and lace-work to the swift and subtle spider. She is the poet, the interpreter of her own grace and ingenuousness, the spinner of the mystery in which her wish to please arrays itself. All the talent she

SIMPLE BEAUTY 145

expends in her effort to equal man in the other arts, is never worth the spirit and conception wrought out through a bit of stuff in her skillful hands.

"Well, I wish that this art were more honored than it is. As education should consist in thinking with one's mind, feeling with one's heart, expressing the little personalities of the inmost, invisible *I*, — which on the contrary are repressed, leveled down by conformity, — I would that the young girl in her novitiate of womanhood, the future mother, might early become the little exponent of this art of the toilet, her own dressmaker in short — she who one day shall make the dresses of her children. But with the taste and the gift to improvise, to express herself in that masterpiece of feminine personality and skill — *a gown*, without which a woman is no more than a bundle of rags."

The dress you have made for yourself is almost always the most becoming, and, however that may be, it is the one that pleases you most. Women of leisure too often forget this; working women, also, in city and country alike. Since these last are costumed by dressmakers and milliners, in very doubtful imitation of the modish world, grace has almost

146 THE SIMPLE LIFE

disappeared from their dress. And has anything more surely the gift to please than the fresh apparition of a young working girl or a daughter of the fields, wearing the costume of her country, and beautiful from her simplicity alone?

These same reflections might be applied to the fashion of decorating and arranging our houses. If there are toilettes which reveal an entire conception of life, hats that are poems, knots of ribbon that are veritable works of art, so there are interiors which after their manner speak to the mind. Why, under pretext of decorating our homes, do we destroy that personal character which always has such value? Why have our sleeping-rooms conform to those of hotels, our reception-rooms to waiting-rooms, by making predominant a uniform type of official beauty?

What a pity to go through the houses of a city, the cities of a country, the countries of a vast continent, and encounter everywhere certain forms, identical, inevitable, exasperating by their repetition! How esthetics would gain by more simplicity! Instead of this luxury in job lots, all these decorations, pretentious but vapid from iteration, we should have an infinite variety; happy improvisations would

SIMPLE BEAUTY 147

strike our eyes, the unexpected in a thousand forms would rejoice our hearts, and we should rediscover the secret of impressing on a drapery or a piece of furniture that stamp of human personality which makes certain antiques priceless.

Let us pass at last to things simpler still; I mean the little details of housekeeping which many young people of our day find so unpoetical. Their contempt for material things, for the humble cares a house demands, arises from a confusion very common but none the less unfortunate, which comes from the belief that beauty and poetry are within some things, while others lack them; that some occupations are distinguished and agreeable, such as cultivating letters, playing the harp; and that others are menial and disagreeable, like blacking shoes, sweeping, and watching the pot boil. Childish error! Neither harp nor broom has anything to do with it; all depends on the hand in which they rest and the spirit that moves it. Poetry is not in things, it is in us. It must be impressed on objects from without, as the sculptor impresses his dream on the marble. If our life and our occupations remain too often without charm, in spite of any outward distinction they may have, it is because we have

148   THE SIMPLE LIFE

not known how to put anything into them. The height of art is to make the inert live, and to tame the savage. I would have our young girls apply themselves to the development of the truly feminine art of giving a soul to things which have none. The triumph of woman's charm is in that work. Only a woman knows how to put into a home that indefinable something whose virtue has made the poet say, "The housetop rejoices and is glad." They say there are no such things as fairies, or that there are fairies no longer, but they know not what they say. The original of the fairies sung by poets was found, and is still, among those amiable mortals who knead bread with energy, mend rents with cheerfulness, nurse the sick with smiles, put witchery into a ribbon and genius into a stew.

IT is indisputable that the culture of the fine arts has something refining about it, and that our thoughts and acts are in the end impregnated with that which strikes our eyes. But the exercise of the arts and the contemplation of their products is a restricted privilege. It is not given to everyone to possess, to comprehend or to create fine things. Yet there is a kind of ministering beauty

SIMPLE BEAUTY 149

which may make its way everywhere — the beauty
which springs from the hands of our wives and
daughters. Without it, what is the most richly
decorated house? A dead dwelling-place. With
it the barest home has life and brightness. Among
the forces capable of transforming the will and
increasing happiness, there is perhaps none in more
universal use than this beauty. It knows how to
shape itself by means of the crudest tools, in the
midst of the greatest difficulties. When the dwelling is cramped, the purse limited, the table modest,
a woman who has the gift, finds a way to make order,
fitness and convenience reign in her house. She
puts care and art into everything she undertakes.
To do well what one has to do is not in her eyes
the privilege of the rich, but the right of all. That
is her aim, and she knows how to give her home
a dignity and an attractiveness that the dwellings of
princes, if everything is left to mercenaries, cannot
possess.

Thus understood, life quickly shows itself rich in
hidden beauties, in attractions and satisfactions close
at hand. To be one's self, to realize in one's
natural place the kind of beauty which is fitting
there — this is the ideal. How the mission of

150   THE SIMPLE LIFE

woman broadens and deepens in significance when
it is summed up in this : to put a soul into the in-
animate, and to give to this gracious spirit of things
those subtle and winsome outward manifestations
to which the most brutish of human beings is sensible. Is not this better than to covet what one
has not, and to give one's self up to longings for a
poor imitation of others' finery ?

XII

PRIDE AND SIMPLICITY IN THE INTER-COURSE OF MEN

IT would perhaps be difficult to find a more convincing example than pride to show that the obstacles to a better, stronger, serener life are rather in us than in circumstances. The diversity, and more than that, the contrasts in social conditions give rise inevitably to all sorts of conflicts. Yet in spite of this how greatly would social relations be simplified, if we put another spirit into mapping out our plan of outward necessities! Be well persuaded that it is not primarily differences of class and occupation, differences in the outward manifestations of their destinies, which embroil men. If such were the case, we should find an idyllic peace reigning among colleagues, and all those whose interests and lot are virtually equivalent. On the contrary, as everyone knows, the most violent shocks come when equal meets equal, and there is no war worse than civil war.

152 THE SIMPLE LIFE

But that which above all things else hinders men from good understanding, is pride. It makes a man a hedgehog, wounding everyone he touches. Let us speak first of the pride of the great.

What offends me in this rich man passing in his carriage, is not his equipage, his dress, or the number and splendor of his retinue : it is his contempt. That he possesses a great fortune does not disturb me, unless I am badly disposed : but that he splashes me with mud, drives over my body, shows by his whole attitude that I count for nothing in his eyes because I am not rich like himself — this is what disturbs me, and righteously. He heaps suffering upon me needlessly. He humiliates and insults me gratuitously. It is not what is vulgar within me, but what is noblest that asserts itself in the face of this offensive pride. Do not accuse me of envy; I feel none; it is my manhood that is wounded. We need not search far to illustrate these ideas. Every man of any acquaintance with life has had numerous experiences which will justify our dictum in his eyes. In certain communities devoted to material interests, the pride of wealth dominates to such a degree that men are quoted like values in the stock market. The esteem in

PRIDE AND SIMPLICITY   153

which a man is held is proportionate to the contents of his strong box. Here "Society" is made up of big fortunes, the middle class of medium fortunes. Then come people who have little, then those who have nothing. All intercourse is regulated by this principle. And the relatively rich man who has shown his disdain for those less opulent, is crushed in turn by the contempt of his superiors in fortune. So the madness of comparison rages from the summit to the base. Such an atmosphere is ready to perfection for the nurture of the worst feeling; yet it is not wealth, but the spirit of the wealthy that must be arraigned.

Many rich men are free from this gross conception — especially is this true of those who from father to son are accustomed to ease — yet they sometimes forget that there is a certain delicacy in not making contrasts too marked. Suppose there is no wrong in enjoying a large superfluity : is it indispensable to display it, to wound the eyes of those who lack necessities, to flaunt one's magnificence at the doors of poverty? Good taste and a sort of modesty always hinder a well man from talking of his fine appetite, his sound sleep, his exuberance of spirits, in the presence of one dying of consumption.

154 THE SIMPLE LIFE

Many of the rich do not exercise this tact, and so are greatly wanting in pity and discretion. Are they not unreasonable to complain of envy, after having done everything to provoke it?

But the greatest lack is that want of discernment which leads men to ground their pride in their fortune. To begin with, it is a childish confusion of thought to consider wealth as a personal quality; it would be hard to find a more ingenuous fashion of deceiving one's self as to the relative value of the container and the thing contained. I have no wish to dwell on this question: it is too painful. And yet one cannot resist saying to those concerned: "Take care, do not confound what you possess with what you are. Go learn to know the under side of worldly splendor, that you may feel its moral misery and its puerility." The traps pride sets for us are too ridiculous. We should distrust association with a thing that make us hateful to our neighbors and robs us of clearness of vision.

He who yields to the pride of riches, forgets this other point, the most important of all — that possession is a public trust. Without doubt, individual wealth is as legitimate as individual existence and liberty. These things are inseparable, and it is a

PRIDE AND SIMPLICITY   155

dream pregnant with dangers that offers battle to
such fundamentals of life.   But the individual
touches society at every point, and all he does
should be done with the whole in view.   Possession,
then, is less a privilege of which to be proud than a
charge whose gravity should be felt.   As there is an
apprenticeship, often very difficult to serve, for the
exercise of every social office, so this profession we
call wealth demands an apprenticeship.   To know
how to be rich is an art, and one of the least easy of
arts to master.   Most people, rich and poor alike,
imagine that in opulence one has nothing to do but
to take life easy.   That is why so few men know how
to be rich.   In the hands of too many, wealth, according to the genial and redoubtable comparison of
Luther, is like a harp in the hoofs of an ass.   They
have no idea of the manner of its use.

So when we encounter a man at once rich and
simple, that is to say, who considers his wealth as a
means of fulfilling his mission in the world, we
should offer him our homage, for he is surely mark-
worthy.   He has surmounted obstacles, borne trials,
and triumphed in temptations both gross and subtle.
He does not fail to discriminate between the contents of his pocketbook and the contents of his

156   THE SIMPLE LIFE

head or heart, and he does not estimate his fellow-men in figures. His exceptional position, instead of exalting him, makes him humble, for he is very sensible of how far he falls short of reaching the level of his duty. He has remained a man — that says it all. He is accessible, helpful, and far from making of his wealth a barrier to separate him from other men, he makes it a means for coming nearer and nearer to them. Although the profession of riches has been so dishonored by the selfish and the proud, such a man as this always makes his worth felt by everyone not devoid of a sense of justice. Each of us who comes in contact with him and sees him live, is forced to look within and ask himself the question, "What would become of me in such a situation? Should I keep this modesty, this naturalness, this uprightness which uses its own as though it belonged to others?" So long as there is a human society in the world, so long as there are bitterly conflicting interests, so long as envy and egoism exist on the earth, nothing will be worthier of honor than wealth permeated by the spirit of simplicity. And it will do more than make itself forgiven; it will make itself beloved.

PRIDE AND SIMPLICITY 157

MORE dangerous than pride inspired by wealth is that inspired by power, and I mean by the word every prerogative that one man has over another, be it unlimited or restricted. I see no means of preventing the existence in the world of men of unequal authority. Every organism supposes a hierarchy of powers — we shall never escape from that law. But I fear that if the love of power is so widespread, the spirit of power is almost impossible to find. From wrong understanding and misuse of it, those who keep even a fraction of authority almost everywhere succeed in compromising it.

Power exercises a great influence over him who holds it. A head must be very well balanced not to be disturbed by it. The sort of dementia which took possession of the Roman emperors in the time of their world-wide rule, is a universal malady whose symptoms belong to all times. In every man there sleeps a tyrant, awaiting only a favorable occasion for waking. Now the tyrant is the worst enemy of authority, because he furnishes us its intolerable caricature, whence come a multitude of social complications, collisions and hatreds. Every man who says to those dependent on him : " Do

158 THE SIMPLE LIFE

this because it is my will and pleasure," does ill.
There is within each one of us something that in-
vites us to resist personal power, and this something is very respectable. For at bottom we are
equal, and there is no one who has the right to exact obedience from me because he is he and I am
I : if he does so, his command degrades me, and I
have no right to suffer myself to be degraded.

One must have lived in schools, in work-shops, in
the army, in Government offices, he must have
closely followed the relations between masters and
servants, have observed a little everywhere where
the supremacy of man exercises itself over man, to
form any idea of the injury done by those who use
power arrogantly. Of every free soul they make
a slave soul, which is to say the soul of a rebel.
And it appears that this result, with its social dis-
aster, is most certain when he who commands is
least removed from the station of him who obeys.
The most implacable tyrant is the tyrant himself
under authority. Foremen and overseers put more
violence into their dealings than superintendents
and employers. The corporal is generally harsher
than the colonel. In certain families where madam
has not much more education than her maid, the

PRIDE AND SIMPLICITY 159

relations between them are those of the convict and his warder. And woe everywhere to him who falls into the hands of a subaltern drunk with his authority!

We forget that the first duty of him who exercises power is humility. Haughtiness is not authority. It is not we who are the law; the law is over our heads. We only interpret it, but to make it valid in the eyes of others, we must first be subject to it ourselves. To command and to obey in the society of men, are after all but two forms of the same virtue — voluntary servitude. If you are not obeyed, it is generally because you have not yourself obeyed first.

The secret of moral ascendancy rests with those who rule with simplicity. They soften by the spirit the harshness of the fact. Their authority is not in shoulder-straps, titles or disciplinary measures. They make use of neither ferule nor threats, yet they achieve everything. Why? Because we feel that they are themselves ready for everything. That which confers upon a man the right to demand of another the sacrifice of his time, his money, his passions, even his life, is not only that he is resolved upon all these sacrifices himself, but

160   THE SIMPLE LIFE

that he has made them in advance. In the command of a man animated by this spirit of renunciation, there is a mysterious force which communicates itself to him who is to obey, and helps him do his duty.

In all the provinces of human activity there are chiefs who inspire, strengthen, magnetize their soldiers: under their direction the troops do prodigies. With them one feels himself capable of any effort, ready to go through fire, as the saying has it; and if he goes, it is with enthusiasm.

BUT the pride of the exalted is not the only pride; there is also the pride of the humble — this arrogance of underlings, fit pendant to that of the great. The root of these two prides is the same. It is not alone that lofty and imperious being, the man who says, "I am the law," that provokes insurrection by his very attitude; it is also that pig-headed subaltern who will not admit that there is anything beyond his knowledge.

There are really many people who find all superiority irritating. For them, every piece of advice is an offense, every criticism an imposition, every

PRIDE AND SIMPLICITY 161

order an outrage on their liberty. They would not know how to submit to rule. To respect anything or anybody would seem to them a mental aberration. They say to people after their fashion : "Beyond us there is nothing."

To the family of the proud belong also those difficult and supersensitive people who in humble life find that their superiors never do them fitting honor, whom the best and most kindly do not succeed in satisfying, and who go about their duties with the air of a martyr. At bottom these disaffected minds have too much misplaced self-respect. They do not know how to fill their place simply, but complicate their life and that of others by unreasonable demands and morbid suspicions.

When one takes the trouble to study men at short range, he is surprised to find that pride has so many lurking-places among those who are by common consent called the humble. So powerful is this vice, that it arrives at forming round those who live in the most modest circumstances a wall which isolates them from their neighbors. There they are, intrenched, barricaded with their ambitions and their contempts, as inaccessible as the powerful of earth behind their aristocratic prejudices. Obscure

162　THE SIMPLE LIFE

or illustrious, pride wraps itself in its dark royalty of enmity to the human race. It is the same in misery and in high places — solitary and impotent, on guard against everybody, embroiling everything. And the last word about it is always this: If there is so much hostility and hatred between different classes of men, it is due less to exterior conditions than to an interior fatality. Conflicting interests and differences of situation dig ditches between us, it is true, but pride transforms the ditches into gulfs, and in reality it is pride alone which cries from brink to brink: "There is nothing in common between you and us."

WE have not finished with pride, but it is impossible to picture it under all its forms. I feel most resentful against it when it meddles with knowledge and appropriates that. We owe our knowledge to our fellows, as we do our riches and power. It is a social force which ought to be of service to everybody, and it can only be so when those who know remain sympathetically near to those who know not. When knowledge is turned into a tool for ambition, it destroys itself.

PRIDE AND SIMPLICITY 163

And what shall we say of the pride of good men ? for it exists, and makes even virtue hateful. The just who repent them of the evil others do, remain in brotherhood and social rectitude. But the just who despise others for their faults and misdeeds, cut themselves off from humanity, and their goodness, descended to the rank of an ornament for their vanity, becomes like those riches which kindness does not inform, like authority untempered by the spirit of obedience. Like proud wealth and arrogant power, supercilious virtue also is detestable. It fosters in man traits and an attitude provocative of I know not what. The sight of it repels instead of attracting, and those whom it deigns to distinguish with its benefits feel as though they had been slapped in the face.

To resume and conclude, it is an error to think that our advantages, whatever they are, should be put to the service of our vanity. Each of them constitutes for him who enjoys it an obligation and not a reason for vainglory. Material wealth, power, knowledge, gifts of the heart and mind, become so much cause for discord when they serve to nourish pride. They remain beneficent only so long as they are the source of modesty in those who possess them.

164 THE SIMPLE LIFE

Let us be humble if we have great possessions, for that proves that we are great debtors : all that a man has he owes to someone, and are we sure of being able to pay our debts ?

Let us be humble if we sit in high places and hold the fate of others in our hands ; for no clear-sighted man can fail to be sensible of unfitness for so grave a rôle.

Let us be humble if we have much knowledge, for it only serves to better show the vastness of the unknown, and to compare the little we have discovered for ourselves with the amplitude of that which we owe to the pains of others.

And, above all, let us be humble if we are virtuous, since no one should be more sensible of his defects than he whose conscience is illumined, and since he more than anyone else should feel the need of charity toward evil-doers, even of suffering in their stead.

"AND what about the necessary distinctions in life?" someone may ask. "As a result of your simplifications, are you not going to destroy that sense of the difference between men which must be maintained if society exists at all ?"

PRIDE AND SIMPLICITY 165

I have no mind to suppress distinctions and differences. But I think that what distinguishes a man is not found in his social rank, his occupation, his dress or his fortune, but solely in himself. More than any other our own age has pricked the vain bubble of purely outward greatness. To be somebody at present, it does not suffice to wear the mantle of an emperor or a royal crown : what honor is there in wielding power through gold lace, a coat of arms or a ribbon? Not that visible signs are to be despised ; they have their meaning and use, but on condition that they cover something and not a vacuum. The moment they cease to stand for realities, they become useless and dangerous. The only true distinction is superior worth. If you would have social rank duly respected, you must begin by being worthy of the rank that is your own ; otherwise you help to bring it into hatred and contempt. It is unhappily too true that respect is diminishing among us, and it certainly is not from a lack of lines drawn round those who wish to be respected. The root of the evil is in the mistaken idea that high station exempts him who holds it from observing the common obligations of life. As we rise, we believe that we free ourselves from the law, forgetting

166 THE SIMPLE LIFE

that the spirit of obedience and humility should grow with our possessions and power. So it comes about that those who demand the most homage make the least effort to merit the homage they demand. This is why respect is diminishing.

The sole distinction necessary is the wish to become better. The man who strives to be better becomes more humble, more approachable, more friendly even with those who owe him allegiance. But as he gains by being better known, he loses nothing in distinction, and he reaps the more respect in that he has sown the less pride.

XIII

THE EDUCATION FOR SIMPLICITY

THE simple life being above all else the product of a direction of mind, it is natural that education should have much to do with it.

In general but two methods of rearing children are practiced : the first is to bring them up for ourselves ; the second, to bring them up for themselves.

In the first case the child is looked upon as a complement of the parents : he is part of their property, occupies a place among their possessions. Sometimes this place is the highest, especially when the parents value the life of the affections. Again, where material interests rule, the child holds second, third, or even the last place. In any case he is a nobody. While he is young, he gravitates round his parents, not only by obedience, which is right, but by the subordination of all his originality, all his being. As he grows older, this subordination

168   THE SIMPLE LIFE

becomes a veritable confiscation, extending to his ideas, his feelings, everything. His minority becomes perpetual. Instead of slowly evolving into independence, the man advances into slavery. He is what he is permitted to be, what his father's business, religious beliefs, political opinions or esthetic tastes require him to be. He will think, speak, act, and marry according to the understanding and limits of the paternal absolutism. This family tyranny may be exercised by people with no strength of character. It is only necessary for them to be convinced that good order requires the child to be the property of the parents. In default of mental force, they possess themselves of him by other means — by sighs, supplications, or base seductions. If they cannot fetter him, they snare his feet in traps. But that he should live in them, through them, for them, is the only thing admissible.

Education of this sort is not the practice of families only, but also of great social organizations whose chief educational function consists in putting a strong hand on every new-comer, in order to fit him, in the most iron-bound fashion, into existing forms. It is the attenuation, pulverization and as-

EDUCATION FOR SIMPLICITY 169

similation of the individual in a social body, be it theocratic, communistic, or simply bureaucratic and routinary. Looked at from without, a like system seems the ideal of simplicity in education. Its processes, in fact, are absolutely simplistic, and if a man were not somebody, if he were only a sample of the race, this would be the perfect education. As all wild beasts, all fish and insects of the same genus and species have the same markings, so we should all be identical, having the same tastes, the same language, the same beliefs, the same tendencies. But man is not simply a specimen of the race, and for that reason this sort of education is far from being simple in its results. Men so vary from one another, that numberless methods have to be invented to repress, stupefy, and extinguish individual thought. And one never arrives at it then but in part, a fact which is continually deranging everything. At each moment, by some fissure, some interior force of initiative is making a violent way to the light, producing explosions, upheavals, all sorts of grave disorders. And where there are no outward manifestations, the evil lies dormant ; beneath apparent order are hidden dumb revolt, flaws made by an abnormal existence, apathy, death.

170 THE SIMPLE LIFE

The system is evil which produces such fruit, and however simple it may appear, in reality it brings forth all possible complications.

THE other system is the extreme opposite, that of bringing up children for themselves. The rôles are reversed: the parents are there for the child. No sooner is he born than he becomes the center. White-headed grandfather and stalwart father bow before these curls. His lisping is their law. A sign from him suffices. If he cries in the night, no fatigue is of account, the whole household must be roused. The new-comer is not long in discovering his omnipotence, and before he can walk he is drunken with it. As he grows older all this deepens and broadens. Parents, grandparents, servants, teachers, everybody is at his command. He accepts the homage and even the immolation of his neighbor: he treats like a rebellious subject anyone who does not step out of his path. There is only himself. He is the unique, the perfect, the infallible. Too late it is perceived that all this has been evolving a master; and what a master! forgetful of sacrifices, without respect, even pity. He no longer has any regard for those to whom he

EDUCATION FOR SIMPLICITY 171

owes everything, and he goes through life without law or check.

This education, too, has its social counterpart. It flourishes wherever the past does not count, where history begins with the living, where there is no tradition, no discipline, no reverence; where those who know the least make the most noise; where those who stand for public order are alarmed by every chance comer whose power lies in his making a great outcry and respecting nothing. It insures the reign of transitory passion, the triumph of the inferior will. I compare these two educations — one, the exaltation of the environment, the other of the individual; one the absolutism of tradition, the other the tyranny of the new — and I find them equally baneful. But the most disastrous of all is the combination of the two, which produces human beings half-automatons, half-despots, forever vacillating between the spirit of a sheep and the spirit of revolt or domination.

Children should be educated neither for themselves nor for their parents: for man is no more designed to be a personage than a specimen. They should be educated for life. The aim of their education is to aid them to become active members of

172 THE SIMPLE LIFE

humanity, brotherly forces, free servants of the civil organization. To follow a method of education inspired by any other principle, is to complicate life, deform it, sow the seeds of all disorders.

When we would sum up in a phrase the destiny of the child, the word future springs to our lips. The child is the future. This word says all — the sufferings of the past, the stress of to-day, hope. But when the education of the child begins, he is incapable of estimating the reach of this word; for he is held by impressions of the present. Who then shall give him the first enlightenment and put him in the way he should go? The parents, the teachers. And with very little reflection they perceive that their work does not interest simply themselves and the child, but that they represent and administer impersonal powers and interests. The child should continually appear to them as a future citizen. With this ruling idea, they will take thought for two things that complement each other — for the initial and personal force which is germinating in the child, and for the social destination of this force. At no moment of their direction over him can they forget that this little being confided to their care must become *himself*

EDUCATION FOR SIMPLICITY 173

and *a brother*. These two conditions, far from excluding each other, never exist apart. It is impossible to be brotherly, to love, to give one's self, unless one is master of himself; and reciprocally, none can possess himself, comprehend his own individual being, until he has first made his way through the outward accidents of his existence, down to the profound springs of life where man feels himself one with other men in all that is most intimately his own.

To aid a child to become himself and a brother it is necessary to protect him against the violent and destructive action of the forces of disorder. These forces are exterior and interior. Every child is menaced from without not only by material dangers but by the meddlesomeness of alien wills; and from within, by an exaggerated idea of his own personality and all the fancies it breeds. There is a great outward danger which may come from the abuse of power in educators. The right of might finds itself a place in education with extreme facility. To educate another, one must have renounced this right, that is to say, made abnegation of the inferior sentiment of personal importance, which transforms us into the enemies of others, even of our own children. Our authority is beneficent only when it is

174 THE SIMPLE LIFE

inspired by one higher than our own. In this case it is not only salutary, but also indispensable, and becomes in its turn the best guarantee against the greater peril which threatens the child from within — that of exaggerating his own importance. At the beginning of life the vividness of personal impressions is so great, that to establish an equilibrium, they must be submitted to the gentle influence of a calm and superior will. The true quality of the office of educator is to represent this will to the child, in a manner as continuous and as disinterested as possible. Educators, then, stand for all that is to be respected in the world. They give to the child impressions of that which precedes it, outruns it, envelops it: but they do not crush it; on the contrary, their will and all the influence they transmit, become elements nutritive of its native energy. Such use of authority as this, cultivates that fruitful obedience out of which free souls are born. The purely personal authority of parents, masters and institutions is to the child like the brushwood beneath which the young plant withers and dies. Impersonal authority, the authority of a man who has first submitted himself to the time-honored realities before which he wishes the

EDUCATION FOR SIMPLICITY 175

individual fancy of the child to bend, resembles pure and luminous air. True it has an activity, and influences us in its manner, but it nourishes our individuality and gives it firmness and stability. Without this authority there is no education. To watch, to guide, to keep a firm hand — such is the function of the educator. He should appear to the child not like a barrier of whims, which, if need be, one may clear, provided the leap be proportioned to the height of the obstacle; but like a transparent wall through which may be seen unchanging realities, laws, limits, and truths against which no action is possible. Thus arises respect, which is the faculty of conceiving something greater than ourselves — respect, which broadens us and frees us by making us more modest. This is the law of education for simplicity. It may be summed up in these words: to make *free* and *reverential* men, who shall be *individual* and *fraternal*.

L ET us draw from this principle some practical applications.

From the very fact that the child is the future, he must be linked to the past by piety. We owe it to him to clothe tradition in the forms

176   THE SIMPLE LIFE

most practical and most fit to create a deep impression : whence the exceptional place that should be given in education to the ancients, to the cult of remembrance of the past, and by extension, to the history of the domestic rooftree. Above all do we fulfil a duty toward our children when we give the place of honor to the grandparents. Nothing speaks to a child with so much force, or so well develops his modesty, as to see his father and mother, on all occasions, preserve toward an old grandfather, often infirm, an attitude of respect. It is a perpetual object lesson that is irresistible. That it may have its full force, it is necessary for a tacit understanding to obtain among all the grown-up members of the family. To the child's eyes they must all be in league, held to mutual respect and understanding, under penalty of compromising their educational authority. And in their number must be counted the servants. Servants are big people, and the same sentiment of respect is injured in the child's disregard of them as in his disregard of his father or grandfather. The moment he addresses an impolite or arrogant word to a person older than himself, he strays from the path that a child ought never to quit ; and if only occasionally the parents

EDUCATION FOR SIMPLICITY 177

neglect to point this out, they will soon perceive by his conduct toward themselves, that the enemy has found entrance to his heart.

We mistake if we think that a child is naturally alien to respect, basing this opinion on the very numerous examples of irreverence which he offers us. Respect is for the child a fundamental need. His moral being feeds on it. The child aspires confusedly to revere and admire something. But when advantage is not taken of this aspiration, it gets corrupted or lost. By our lack of cohesion and mutual deference, we, the grown-ups, discredit daily in the child's eyes our own cause and that of everything worthy of respect. We inoculate in him a bad spirit whose effects then turn against us.

This pitiful truth nowhere appears with more force than in the relations between masters and servants, as we have made them. Our social errors, our want of simplicity and kindness, all fall back upon the heads of our children. There are certainly few people of the middle classes who understand that it is better to part with many thousands of dollars than to lead their children to lose respect for servants, who represent in our households the

178 THE SIMPLE LIFE

humble. Yet nothing is truer. Maintain as strictly as you will conventions and distances, — that demarkation of social frontiers which permits each one to remain in his place and to observe the law of differences. That is a good thing, I am persuaded, but on condition of never forgetting that those who serve us are men and women like ourselves. You require of your domestics certain formulas of speech and certain attitudes, outward evidence of the respect they owe you. Do you also teach your children and use yourselves manners toward your servants which show them that you respect their dignity as individuals, as you desire them to respect yours? Here we have continually in our homes an excellent ground for experiment in the practice of that mutual respect which is one of the essential conditions of social sanity. I fear we profit by it too little. We do not fail to exact respect, but we fail to give it. So it is most frequently the case that we get only hypocrisy and this supplementary result, all unexpected, — the cultivation of pride in our children. These two factors combined heap up great difficulties for that future which we ought to be safeguarding. I am right then in saying that the day when by your own practices you have

EDUCATION FOR SIMPLICITY   179

brought about the lessening of respect in your children, you have suffered a sensible loss.

Why should I not say it? It seems to me that the greater part of us labor for this loss. On all sides, in almost every social rank, I notice that a pretty bad spirit is fostered in children, a spirit of reciprocal contempt. Here, those who have calloused hands and working-clothes are disdained; there, it is all who do not wear blue jeans. Children educated in this spirit make sad fellow-citizens. There is in all this the want of that simplicity which makes it possible for men of good intentions, of however diverse social standing, to collaborate without any friction arising from the conventional distance that separates them.

If the spirit of caste causes the loss of respect, partisanship, of whatever sort, is quite as productive of it. In certain quarters children are brought up in such fashion that they respect but one country — their own; one system of government — that of their parents and masters; one religion — that which they have been taught. Does anyone suppose that in this way men can be shaped who shall respect country, religion and law? Is this a proper respect — this respect which does not extend

180 THE SIMPLE LIFE

beyond what touches and belongs to ourselves?
Strange blindness of cliques and coteries, which arrogate to themselves with so much ingenuous complacence the title of schools of respect, and which, outside themselves, respect nothing. In reality they teach : " Country, religion, law — we are all these ! " Such teaching fosters fanaticism, and if fanaticism is not the sole anti-social ferment, it is surely one of the worst and most energetic.

IF simplicity of heart is an essential condition of respect, simplicity of life is its best school. Whatever be the state of your fortune, avoid everything which could make your children think themselves more or better than others. Though your wealth would permit you to dress them richly, remember the evil you might do in exciting their vanity. Preserve them from the evil of believing that to be elegantly dressed suffices for distinction, and above all do not carelessly increase by their clothes and their habits of life, the distance which already separates them from other children : dress them simply. And if, on the contrary, it would be necessary for you to economize to give your children the pleasure of fine clothes, I

EDUCATION FOR SIMPLICITY 181

would that I might dispose you to reserve your spirit of sacrifice for a better cause. You risk seeing it illy recompensed. You dissipate your money when it would much better avail to save it for serious needs, and you prepare for yourself, later on, a harvest of ingratitude. How dangerous it is to accustom your sons and daughters to a style of living beyond your means and theirs! In the first place, it is very bad for your purse; in the second place it develops a contemptuous spirit in the very bosom of the family. If you dress your children like little lords, and give them to understand that they are superior to you, is it astonishing if they end by disdaining you ? You will have nourished at your table the declassed — a product which costs dear and is worthless.

Any fashion of instructing children whose most evident result is to lead them to despise their parents and the customs and activities among which they have grown up, is a calamity. It is effective for nothing but to produce a legion of malcontents, with hearts totally estranged from their origin, their race, their natural interests — everything, in short, that makes the fundamental fabric of a man. Once detached from the vigorous stock which produced them, the wind of their restless ambition drives

182   THE SIMPLE LIFE

them over the earth, like dead leaves that will in the end be heaped up to ferment and rot together.

Nature does not proceed by leaps and bounds, but by an evolution slow and certain. In preparing a career for our children, let us imitate her. Let us not confound progress and advancement with those violent exercises called somersaults. Let us not so bring up our children that they will come to despise work and the aspirations and simple spirit of their fathers: let us not expose them to the temptation of being ashamed of our poverty if they themselves come to fortune. A society is indeed diseased when the sons of peasants begin to feel disgust for the fields, when the sons of sailors desert the sea, when the daughters of workingmen, in the hope of being taken for heiresses, prefer to walk the streets alone rather than beside their honest parents. A society is healthy, on the contrary, when each of its members applies himself to doing very nearly what his parents have done before him, but doing it better, and, looking to future elevation, is content first to fulfill conscientiously more modest duties.*

---

* This would be the place to speak of work in general, and of its tonic effect upon education. But I have discussed the subject in my books *Justice, Jeunesse,* and *Vaillance.* I must limit myself to referring the reader to them.

EDUCATION FOR SIMPLICITY 183

EDUCATION should make independent men. If you wish to train your children for liberty, bring them up simply, and do not for a moment fear that in so doing you are putting obstacles in the way of their happiness. It will be quite the contrary. The more costly toys a child has, the more feasts and curious entertainments, the less is he amused.

In this there is a sure sign. Let us be temperate in our methods of entertaining youth, and especially let us not thoughtlessly create for them artificial needs. Food, dress, nursery, amusements — let all these be as natural and simple as possible. With the idea of making life pleasant for their children, some parents bring them up in habits of gormandizing and idleness, accustom them to sensations not meant for their age, multiply their parties and entertainments. Sorry gifts these! In place of a free man, you are making a slave. Gorged with luxury, he tires of it in time; and yet when for one reason or another his pleasures fail him, he will be miserable, and you with him: and what is worse, perhaps in some capital encounter of life, you will be ready — you and he together — to sacrifice manly dignity, truth, and duty, from sheer sloth.

184 THE SIMPLE LIFE

Let us bring up our children simply, I had almost said rudely. Let us entice them to exercise that gives them endurance — even to privations. Let them belong to those who are better trained to fatigue and the earth for a bed than to the comforts of the table and couches of luxury. So we shall make men of them, independent and staunch, who may be counted on, who will not sell themselves for pottage, and who will have withal the faculty of being happy.

A too easy life brings with it a sort of lassitude in vital energy. One becomes blasé, disillusioned, an old young man, past being diverted. How many young people are in this state! Upon them have been deposited, like a sort of mold, the traces of our decrepitude, our skepticism, our vices, and the bad habits they have contracted in our company. What reflections upon ourselves these youths weary of life force us to make! What announcements are graven on their brows!

These shadows say to us by contrast that happiness lies in a life true, active, spontaneous, ungalled by the yoke of the passions, of unnatural needs, of unhealthy stimulus; keeping intact the physical faculty of enjoying the light of day and the air we

EDUCATION FOR SIMPLICITY 185

breathe, and in the heart, the capacity to thrill with the love of all that is generous, simple and fine.

THE artificial life engenders artificial thought, and a speech little sure of itself. Normal habits, deep impressions, the ordinary contact with reality, bring frankness with them. Falsehood is the vice of a slave, the refuge of the cowardly and weak. He who is free and strong is unflinching in speech. We should encourage in our children the hardihood to speak frankly. What do we ordinarily do ? We trample on natural disposition, level it down to the uniformity which for the crowd is synonymous with good form. To think with one's own mind, feel with one's own heart, express one's own personality — how unconventional, how rustic ! — Oh ! the atrocity of an education which consists in the perpetual muzzling of the only thing that gives any of us his reason for being ! Of how many soul-murders do we become guilty ! Some are struck down with bludgeons, others gently smothered with pillows ! Everything conspires against independence of character. When we are little, people wish us to be dolls or graven images ; when we grow up, they approve of us

186 THE SIMPLE LIFE

on condition that we are like all the rest of the world — automatons : when you have seen one of them you've seen them all. So the lack of originality and initiative is upon us, and platitude and monotony are the distinctions of to-day. Truth can free us from this bondage : let our children be taught to be themselves, to ring clear, without crack or muffle. Make loyalty a need to them, and in their gravest failures, if only they acknowledge them, account it for merit that they have not covered their sin.

To frankness let us add ingenuousness, in our solicitude as educators. Let us have for this comrade of childhood — a trifle uncivilized, it is true, but so gracious and friendly ! — all possible regard. We must not frighten it away : when it has once fled, it so rarely comes back ! Ingenuousness is not simply the sister of truth, the guardian of the individual qualities of each of us ; it is besides a great informing and educating force. I see among us too many practical people, so called, who go about armed with terrifying spectacles and huge shears to ferret out naïve things and clip their wings. They uproot ingenuousness from life, from thought, from education, and pursue it even to the region of

EDUCATION FOR SIMPLICITY 187

dreams. Under pretext of making men of their children, they prevent their being children at all; — as if before the ripe fruit of autumn, flowers did not have to be, and perfumes, and songs of birds, and all the fairy springtime.

I ask indulgence for everything naïve and simple, not alone for the innocent conceits that flutter round the curly heads of children, but also for the legend, the folk song, the tales of the world of marvel and mystery. The sense of the marvellous is in the child the first form of that sense of the infinite without which a man is like a bird deprived of wings. Let us not wean the child from it, but let us guard in him the faculty of rising above what is earthy, so that he may appreciate later on those pure and moving symbols of vanished ages wherein human truth has found forms of expression that our arid logic will never replace.

XIV

CONCLUSION

I THINK I have said enough of the spirit and manifestations of the simple life, to make it evident that there is here a whole forgotten world of strength and beauty. He can make conquest of it who has sufficient energy to detach himself from the fatal rubbish that trammels our days. It will not take him long to perceive that in renouncing some surface satisfactions and childish ambitions, he increases his faculty of happiness and his possibilities of right judgment.

These results concern as much the private as the public life. It is incontestable that in striving against the feverish will to shine, in ceasing to make the satisfaction of our desires the end of our activity, in returning to modest tastes, to the true life, we shall labor for the unity of the family. Another spirit will breath in our homes, creating new customs and an atmosphere more favorable to the education of children. Little by little our boys and

CONCLUSION 189

girls will feel the enticement of ideals at once higher and more realizable. And transformation of the home will in time exercise its influence on public spirit. As the solidity of a wall depends upon the grain of the stones and the consistence of the cement which binds them together, so also the energy of public life depends upon the individual value of men and their power of cohesion. The great desideratum of our time is the culture of the component parts of society, of the individual man. Everything in the present social organism leads us back to this element. In neglecting it we expose ourselves to the loss of the benefits of progress, even to making our most persistent efforts turn to our own hurt. If in the midst of means continually more and more perfected, the workman diminishes in value, of what use are these fine tools at his disposal? By their very excellence to make more evident the faults of him who uses them without discernment or without conscience. The wheelwork of the great modern machine is infinitely delicate. Carelessness, incompetence or corruption may produce here disturbances of far greater gravity than would have threatened the more or less rudimentary organism of **the society of the past.** There is need then of look-

190 THE SIMPLE LIFE

ing to the quality of the individual called upon to contribute in any measure to the workings of this mechanism. This individual should be at once solid and pliable, inspired with the central law of life — to be one's self and fraternal. Everything within us and without us becomes simplified and unified under the influence of this law, which is the same for everybody and by which each one should guide his actions; for our essential interests are not opposing, they are identical. In cultivating the spirit of simplicity, we should arrive, then, at giving to public life a stronger cohesion.

The phenomena of decomposition and destruction that we see there may all be attributed to the same cause, — lack of solidity and cohesion. It will never be possible to say how contrary to social good are the trifling interests of caste, of coterie, of church, the bitter strife for personal welfare, and, by a fatal consequence, how destructive these things are of individual happiness. A society in which each member is preoccupied with his own well-being, is organized disorder. This is all that we learn from the irreconcilable conflicts of our uncompromising egoism.

We too much resemble those people who claim

CONCLUSION 191

the rights of family only to gain advantage from them, not to do honor to the connection. On all rounds of the social ladder we are forever putting forth claims. We all take the ground that we are creditors : no one recognizes the fact that he is a debtor, and our dealings with our fellows consist in inviting them, in tones sometimes amiable, sometimes arrogant, to discharge their indebtedness to us. No good thing is attained in this spirit. For in fact it is the spirit of privilege, that eternal enemy of universal law, that obstacle to brotherly understanding which is ever presenting itself anew.

IN a lecture delivered in 1882, M. Renan said that a nation is "a spiritual family," and he added : "The essential of a nation is that all the individuals should have many things in common, and also that all should have forgotten much." It is important to know what to forget and what to remember, not only in the past, but also in our daily life. Our memories are lumbered with the things that divide us ; the things which unite us slip away. Each of us keeps at the most luminous point of his souvenirs, a lively sense of his secondary quality, his part of agriculturist, day laborer, man of letters,

192   THE SIMPLE LIFE

public officer, proletary, bourgeois, or political or religious sectarian ; but his essential quality, which is to be a son of his country and a man, is relegated to the shade. Scarcely does he keep even a theoretic notion of it. So that what occupies us and determines our actions, is precisely the thing that separates us from others, and there is hardly place for that spirit of unity which is as the soul of a people.

So too do we foster bad feeling in our brothers. Men animated by a spirit of particularism, exclusiveness, and pride, are continually clashing. They cannot meet without rousing afresh the sentiment of division and rivalry. And so there slowly heaps up in their remembrance a stock of reciprocal ill-will, of mistrust, of rancor. All this is bad feeling with its consequences.

It must be rooted out of our midst. Remember, forget ! This we should say to ourselves every morning, in all our relations and affairs. Remember the essential, forget the accessory ! How much better should we discharge our duties as citizens, if high and low were nourished from this spirit ! How easy to cultivate pleasant remembrances in the mind of one's neighbor, by sowing it with kind

CONCLUSION 193

leeds and refraining from procedures of which in spite of himself he is forced to say, with hatred in his heart: " Never in the world will I forget! "

The spirit of simplicity is a great magician. It softens asperities, bridges chasms, draws together hands and hearts. The forms which it takes in the world are infinite in number; but never does it seem to us more admirable than when it shows itself across the fatal barriers of position, interest, or prejudice, overcoming the greatest obstacles, permitting those whom everything seems to separate to understand one another, esteem one another, love one another. This is the true social cement, that goes into the building of a people.

THE END.

CPSIA information can be obtained at www.ICGtesting.com
Printed in the USA
LVOW030528300112

266017LV00001BA/91/A